# presence

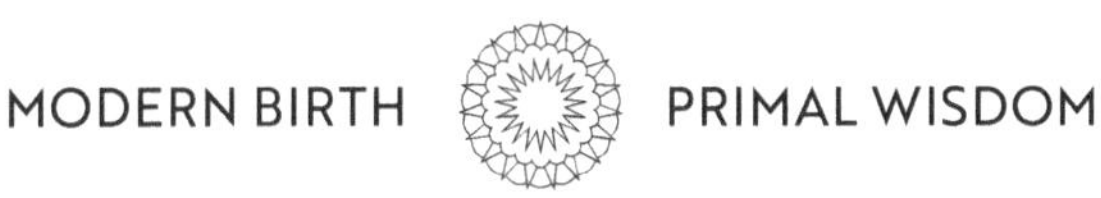


By Margaret McKinney Buxton

PRESENCE
Modern Birth, Primal Wisdom
by Margaret Buxton



This book is a work of nonfiction. The stories, insights, and reflections shared are based on the author's lived experience and professional practice. In all cases where birth stories are shared, details have been changed or generalized to protect the privacy of individuals.



For inquiries, permissions, or speaking requests, visit
DrMargaretBuxton.com

ISBN: 979-8-218-88777-3

Printed on demand. Country of manufacture varies by order fulfillment provider.

Cover design and interior layout by Bella Stern and Studio Delger

First Edition
Published by Margaret H. Buxton
2025

*To my beautiful sisters,*
*with love*

# Contents

## MEDICAL DISCLAIMER

*A Note Before We Begin*

This book is for educational purposes and is not medical advice, nor should it be used for purposes of treatment or diagnosis. While I am a certified nurse midwife with decades of experience, this book is not a substitute for individualized advice, care, treatment, or diagnosis from a qualified healthcare provider.

Every body, every pregnancy, and every birth is different. If you're navigating a medical decision, experiencing symptoms, or have questions about your care, please reach out to your provider or birth team.

The stories, reflections, and insights in this book are meant to support, not replace, your own established clinical care or personal intuition. My hope is that *Presence* helps you feel more grounded, more informed, and more connected as you walk your unique path.

You deserve care that sees you,
listens to you, and meets your needs.

# introduction

**I AM A MIDWIFE.** This permits me to enter intimate, vulnerable places with other humans moving through major life transformations. A midwife is also a magnet for conversation. Learning this about me, people inevitably and effortlessly move to their birth story, drawn toward the meaning-making of their birth journey.

Many midwives can attest to this invitation to listen, and I have had the privilege of hearing incredible stories. Sometimes it's random. I rest in the dentist chair with instruments in my mouth, making affirming sounds, "Uh-huh." Sometimes I have been a chosen care provider, and the telling is a cautionary tale of what they don't want to happen again. Sometimes it's to listen almost as a therapist might, a friend of a friend who "needs to talk to someone" and process something hard. I listen, I nod, my brow crinkles as I wince at the description of traumatic events, and say, "Thank you for sharing this." Other times it's lighter: a dinner party or a girls' night out. I am the trusted recipient of remarkable birth stories, origin stories, and transformation stories.

The telling is important. My primal self knows to sit and be still as I listen, gathering details and inflections, studying their face and body. I know I am on sacred ground, certain they are sharing their story to seek understanding and to affirm an intuitive sense that has already emerged within them. Affirming a woman's intuitive understanding gives her access to her inner strength and power. I also know through these stories, we are inextricably connected. It took years of clinical practice to truly understand the powerful forces at play in the liminal space of labor and birth, but I began to see the themes emerge. Many pieces of a whole.

Our journey through pregnancy, miscarriages, abortions, and birth is far too often isolated. This isolation blocks the reckoning of a full spectrum of emotions. Once a pregnancy ends, it's back to work or life like nothing happened. I knew intuitively, even as a young midwife, the telling of the story was a piece of healing, a piece of the meaning-making. Our stories truly connect us; when we tell them, we realize we're not alone.

Despite our modern scientific advancements, being pregnant, giving birth, and becoming a parent in the 21st century come with many unexpected experiences. Our healthcare system, often primed to care for itself, may leave the birthing family alone to wade through a sea of experiences, many of which can result in a feeling of disempowerment, abandonment, racism, classism, sexism, homophobia, and misogyny. Our culture, far from being birth-positive and inclusive, has left women at times feeling judged, shamed, and isolated on this sacred journey. Birthing families need positive messages, belonging, respect, support, love, and connection.

There's a question hanging in the air for every person facing their fertility. Do I want this? Can I even get pregnant? Are we born as badass mother birthers? I think the answer is yes, but said better as "Yes, and...."

When I listen to birth stories, I often notice the best birth experiences were shaped in small and unexpected ways. It's not that they had it all planned out and perfectly choreographed right down to the color of their toenail polish on the due date. The small and unexpected details that mattered were how they were cared for, who held their hand, how they were listened to, and believed.

The "Yes, and" is this: We thrived as humans because we had people who held space and cared for us in our time of vulnerability. We did this together because we lived in a community and took care of each other; belonging was a part of life. And we know this to be true because it's been studied. It's called primitive gynecology, the origin of midwifery, and the reason our species proliferated[1]. The earliest fossil records show early humans helped each other on this journey to give birth and care for their children. Midwife means "with woman,"

---

[1]Bohannon, C. (2023). Eve: *How the female body drove 200 million years of human evolution*. Alfred A. Knopf.

and in its early and simplest form was the art and practice of presence. You are here because of the power of presence.

Presence is an interesting word; to understand its meaning, think about how we use it.

- Your presence in the room is requested.
- She has such a delightful presence.
- Something about their presence was a little off.

Presence is about bringing energy and intention. It can be something we do for ourselves or receive through our connection to each other. When we "hold space," we are bringing presence. True presence is focused and directed and brings the same kind of energy as what we might find in a flow state. Presence is pausing routine activities to acknowledge something important is happening and giving it your unwavering attention. Where there is a depth of awareness, there is presence. It is noticing your emotions, your body, and your environment. Being able to create this presence for yourself and connect with it in community is an integral part of the journey of pregnancy, birth, and parenting. It seems so simple, but in a distracted and self-involved world, we're losing critical skills around the art of presence.

The question remains: Why did we need help giving birth? Why wasn't it effortless and automatic like it is for so many other species? While evolutionary biology theories abound, I feel comforted that modern midwifery isn't modern at all. It's as old as we are. Social connection and the art of human presence are why we have survived as a species. Yet, here we are in our modern era, able to help in so many ways with medical intervention, but not fully embracing the time-tested ingredient that served us so well for so long: presence.

For almost three decades, I've been a practicing midwife primarily in hospital settings. I've seen the best and worst of what our healthcare system has to offer. But these settings haven't been designed around the critical ingredient of presence, love, and human connection. If you look at it through that lens, you can go as far as to say our system is broken.

Of course, the hospital setting offers so much. We need the wonders of modern medicine and the support of the hospital system when births move into high-risk moments. But this has to exist alongside another truth: We need the connection to our human blueprint, and we need bridges of understanding from our past to our present. We must be present for ourselves, each other, and our communities as we re-remember how to bring love into the birthing room. We can do better. There needs to be a chorus of midwives, doctors, parents, grandparents, and healthcare providers seeking and uplifting a new paradigm, one that honors presence as both necessary and integral to positive birth outcomes.

The purpose of this book is to give you new knowledge and insight that not only better prepares you for your birth or the birth of someone you love, but also gives you a song sheet to join in the chorus. Through this book, you'll gain essential skills, awareness, and understanding of your body's changes, helping you show up more fully each day — for yourself, your baby, and the transformational birth which lies ahead.

There is an inherent paradox: We need each other on the journey, and our physical and metaphysical transformation is unique to ourselves. You need community, and this is a solo journey; and your ability to hold these two truths becomes the foundation of transformation. This is the beginning of that soulful work.

Over the years, I have walked alongside many women on their birth journey. And in my birthing journey, I had the gift of good company and guides. I hope these reflections, insights, and stories will assist you in recognizing your self-worth and in cultivating a supportive community. As you assemble a supportive team of care providers, may you also embrace the family and friends who love and value you throughout this journey. I believe wholeheartedly connecting to a community that is right for you will positively impact your birth. I invite you to open yourself up to this important truth: You need attentive, loving, care-filled support on this journey from pregnancy to childbirth and parenting. This book will connect you to the blueprint and critical tools to do that.

# rites of presence

**THERE IS A RHYTHM TO THIS JOURNEY.** Sitting with people in the liminal space of birth and the raw beginnings of parenthood, I began to see the patterns as themes: joy, power, loss, release, becoming.

These stories, and my own experience as a mother and midwife, led me to a quiet truth: Presence is not something you witness; it is something that happens inside of you. You might recognize this as an inner strength or knowing. This book is not a step-by-step manual. It's a companion. It is an invitation to the moments that rise to meet you. You may be the type to move through this book in a single sitting. You may be the type to set this down and come back to it throughout your pregnancy journey. I encourage you to be reflective. Notice where you are and what you might need.

Yes, birth is a *rite of passage*[2]. But I also believe it's supported, sometimes profoundly, by what I call the *rites of presence*. Rites are defined as *observances, practices*[3]. These aren't ceremonies, but moments. Breath. Safety. Surrender. Receiving. Rites we return to again and again, not just once. Rites that nurture and support our inner knowing and strength.

These rites appear in unexpected places: the moment you ask a question you're afraid to bring to your healthcare provider. The moment your contractions take over, or you decide to stop resisting. The moment you grieve what didn't go the way you planned, but you open yourself anyway.

Presence isn't a goal or a destination. It's taking these moments as they come and making them yours. Finding a rhythm. And like the rhythm of labor, it requires deep trust. You will forget it. You may become distracted. But you can and you will come back to it. That's the work.

These Rites of Presence emerge over and over again throughout the book. They are deeply part of the rite of passage of birth. They are not milestones, nor are they boxes to check. They are tools for cultivating a way of being with the "what is" unfolding. They are foundational to the journey of pregnancy, birth, and parenting. They are tools and a process you'll come back to and cultivate through the lessons in this book.

---

[2]Davis-Floyd, R. (2003). *Birth as an American rite of passage* (2nd ed). University of California Press.

[3]Collins Dictionary. (n.d.). Rite. In *Collins English Dictionary*. Retrieved March 5, 2026, from https://www.collinsdictionary.com/dictionary/english/rite

### REMEMBERING

We are invited to start by returning to what we already know deep in our bodies. Reclaiming the knowledge our culture asked us to forget. Birth, parenting, and transformation are not things to control but ways to connect. And we can start to reconnect and remember this knowledge through our bodies.

### ROOTING

With rooting, you become present to how your body feels by awakening your senses and building a nest around the things that matter to you. You start to ask for what you need. You begin to create a safe space, gather a safe tribe, and from there, presence can emerge.

### RELEASING

Releasing is the letting go of control, of perfection, of certainty. Of who you thought you were. Of the unhelpful inherited cultural ideas you were handed. You do not need to have it all figured out. You start with breath and stay connected to yourself, releasing what you no longer need to hold.

### RECEIVING

Receiving is the best part, the soft landing. The bonding. The moment you are held and the moments you hold. This is the beginning of parenting and also the beginning of a new self. You are not who you were; you are in a state of becoming a new person. And you are not alone.

These four processes sometimes work independently. But they can also work in a flow, allowing you to return to yourself. Some may call this "recentering." But really, it's just a way to settle your internal nervous system and move back toward a place of calm and presence.

Remember the ancient wisdom our bodies already know. Root yourself in the present. Breathe in.

Release control, perfection, and attachment. Breathe out.

Receive the innate love within and the love from those you trust.

None of this may even make sense to you right now, and that's okay. This book will teach you.

This is the beginning of your journey, and not knowing means you might be open to learning. We will spend time together unpacking these ideas and equipping you for the path ahead. **As we move through this journey to welcome new life, you will likely move through these rites again and again. That's the point; we were made to live in these rhythms.**

# origin story

**THE PERSON WHO HELPED ME** understand birth rhythms was the midwife who trained me, Pamela Hunt. "The whole thing is about love, Margaret. It's about bringing love into the room." In her beautiful and simple explanation, she was in touch with our human need for connection and presence, our primitive gynecology. Pamela, a wise and soulful midwife who gave me my start in my career, also helped me enter this world.

I was born on The Farm, one of the largest and most successful American communes in history. The hippies who arrived on The Farm in the early 1970s had robust aspirations to change the world. Those ambitions were actualized by the influence they have had on midwifery in the United States and the world. A massive piece of this influence was the publication of *Spiritual Midwifery*, a groundbreaking book, a collection of stories about home births and a how-to handbook for midwives. No one could have predicted the impact that sharing their stories of natural birth would make. Published in 1975 by one of The Farm's pioneering midwives, Ina May Gaskin, *Spiritual Midwifery* continues to inform and inspire the natural birth movement. The collection of stories chronicling the birth experiences of women and their midwives in the early years of The Farm spurred a countercultural birth revolution. The impact of these stories can still be felt around the world today.

The story of my birth is chronicled in *Spiritual Midwifery*. My mother recounts she and my father were trying to get pregnant. Surrounded by young couples having babies, they were ready. The Farm midwives cared for all of the mothers on The Farm and many more who came there to have their babies, providing prenatal and birth care. When my mother missed her period, she excitedly told Pamela Hunt, one of the founding Farm midwives, who told me about bringing love into the room two decades later. "Check your tits, your nipples will darken if you're pregnant," Pamela said. My mother recounts she looked down her shirt at her braless, changing breasts, and got excited, they were darker! "Come to the clinic next week," Pamela told her, and my mom embarked on a journey to welcome me and later four more sweet souls into her arms at home on The Farm, surrounded by a supportive community.

That's the setting for my own birth story, in a cobbled-together house in the Tennessee woods. It was not a mistake or an accident. It was their plan. My parents had made their way to The Farm a few years earlier. Spiritual-seekers who were looking to be part of something bigger than themselves. Like many young people, the hippie movement that inspired my parents was trying to differentiate itself from their "greatest generation" parents. With the Vietnam War dominating their lived experience, my parents and many others were determined not to go to war. As they watched their political leaders and spiritual heroes being gunned down, they decided to live off the land as vegan pacifists, taking vows of poverty. Part of this movement included the desire to have babies at home, naturally, and to be independent of the medical establishment.

The house where my mother gave birth was called the Adobe. Built in the 1970s with found materials, it was one of just a few actual houses on The Farm. Most of the early members, including my parents, lived in buses or army tents with no bathroom or kitchen. They made do by hauling water from the creek and using outhouses. Resources were scarce, everyone had to do their part to survive, and conditions were not ideal.

Compared to many of the tent dwellings, the Adobe was one of the more "upscale" structures on The Farm with a real kitchen and actual rooms. The loft where I was born was sparse, with a lean-to ladder instead of stairs, and a mattress on the floor in close proximity to the roof line. My parents recount that despite the lack of amenities, they felt lucky not to be in the army tent where they lived and to have a proper shelter to welcome their baby.

On that stormy night, headlamps helped the midwives see my head crowning as my mother breathed heavily in the dark, humid attic. Loud thunder ripped through the June evening, rain pouring down on the tin roof so loudly the midwives' voices were almost inaudible.

They had quite the adventure ahead of them that night: Two mothers were in labor. Upstairs and downstairs they'd go, checking on each birthing mother. Another little girl arrived that evening in June, and I arrived shortly thereafter. The details are chronicled as one of many stories immortalized in *Spiritual Midwifery*, with an image of my chubby little toddler face riding on my father's shoulders to accompany the tale.

My dad said he was walking down the main road of The Farm some months after my birth when Ina May Gaskin stopped in her pickup truck. "Hey, I heard you did a good job at your birth. Would you be willing to write your birth story for me?" she asked. My dad recounts The Farm midwives "walked on water" and the only thing he got out of his mouth that day was, "Sure."

I arrived earthside as a "hard start," my father told me, meaning I didn't cry right away. The midwife's hands I tumbled into that night was catching her first baby, surrounded by her mentors. My midwife brain combs over this fact often. What was she thinking when she saw me pale and limp? How long did it take me to breathe? Did they ventilate my lungs with mouth-to-mouth? How long did I spend in that space? Many years later, I was gifted with more information through the mother who had had her baby in the room below an hour or so before. As she held her newborn girl, she heard the loud cries of my mother — the ecstatic crescendo of birth followed by silence. She was waiting to listen to my cry, and it was disturbingly quiet. She heard my mother's voice in the silence, "Breathe baby…I love you." She remembered saying prayers and then, some time later, heard the sound of my wails.

When it was all over, back to the army tent my parents went with me in the Tennessee summer to bond as a new family, the first baby among many more to come.

The 1970s were an interesting pivot point in history: A generation was rejecting their parents' values, protesting their government, and opening themselves to alternative viewpoints. Their parents gave birth in hospitals during the post WWII era. Mothers were often drugged and separated from their babies. Breastfeeding was shunned, and women were expected to stay isolated in their homes to raise the children. Two decades later, my parents' generation took action: tune in, turn on, and drop out. The Farm was an alternative community that became a refuge for people who wanted to live off the grid and find new ways to be global citizens. A small group of women led by Ina May Gaskin began to attend births, first in buses on a caravan traveling across the country and then in the Tennessee woods. They learned all they could and networked with healthcare professionals for help when needed. Their journey over several decades is well-documented, and the stories are a cultural treasure.

There they were, dirt-poor hippies living and sleeping in buses, ramshackle homes, and tents in the woods. Yet they were having unprecedented rates of health and success giving birth, virtually no cesareans, rare infant mortality, and no maternal mortality[4]. Yes, they were young. They were healthy. There were a few mothers with high-risk factors. Still, the outstanding level of statistical success, with virtually no medical intervention, told a story, too. Positivity, love, and presence were a critical part of the equation.

And so, a positive birth culture was created on The Farm, one in which families were cared for, educated, and nurtured by midwives. Local doctors were called on to help when needed and supported the work of the midwives. Reverence and consciousness were the norm in the birth setting, and each soul's entrance was a celebration.

My dad told me getting "kicked out of my birth" was his greatest fear. This had happened to several of his friends because those same midwives, who he said walked on water, also had the authority to send people out of the room if they believed their energy was blocking a mother's ability to cope or progress. He was so determined not to get kicked out of the birth of his first child that he told me he didn't say *one word* through the birth process and did whatever the midwives told him to. If you knew my dad, you would fully understand what an epic feat this silence and compliance were. But this story perfectly captures how much these young midwives knew. They knew about the art and practice of presence. And apparently, my dad learned quickly too: Get uptight? Get bossy? Get kicked out.

The impact of The Farm midwives continued to grow well after The Farm transitioned away from being a commune, with

---

[4]Duran, A. M. (1992). The safety of home birth: The Farm Study. *American Journal of Public Health*, 82, 450-453.

Ina May continuing to publish books on midwifery and The Farm midwives continuing to have a beautiful practice, with women traveling from all over the world to give birth in this vibrant community.

I feel lucky to have had such close relationships and access to The Farm midwives' stories, insights, and wisdom in my journey to becoming a midwife. Many women worldwide have greatly benefited from their work, and we are all indebted to The Farm midwives who bravely blazed new pathways for becoming midwives and mothers. I imagine those young Farm midwives believed their actions would change the world. They did.

But I am sure they would not have imagined where we are now: one in three babies being born by major surgery, a rising maternal mortality rate, institutional racism still rampant, and a birth culture exchanging connection for convenience.

Most of the women on The Farm were part of the generation that had been delivered in hospitals. It may sound surprising, but birth moved largely into hospitals only in the 1950s, which means while institutionalized birth is a relatively new phenomenon, it is the only one that most people know.

By comparison, midwifery is as old as time. Women have been *with* other women in pregnancy and childbirth from the beginning, bringing the power of presence.

We left The Farm when I was 11 years old, and I was tossed into a culture and a society I had to learn to navigate; it was shocking and shaping. Imagine being in the same state you've always lived in and moving two hours north to a new city, except this new city was utterly foreign to you. Homegrown school to public education, multifamily households to a nuclear family, midwestern plain speak to impossibly hard to understand Southern slang, no exposure to television to constant media access, fresh food from the fields to trips to a sterile grocery store. Being very poor and not realizing it, to being very poor and feeling it, acutely.

Everything in my environment was a discovery, but I wanted to fit in, so I learned how to learn quickly and quietly. I was an eager student, a rule follower, and I had the ability to "read" people and know what they needed. For years, this observant knowing has served me well in the clinical setting and helped me bring presence to the families I cared for. My connection to The Farm and the perspective of my parents and mentors have also stayed with me. At some point, that quiet desire to assimilate to the status quo has given way to bigger and bolder thinking, especially about childbirth, and a willingness to make real change. The kind of real, lasting change that continues the ripples of change started by The Farm midwives.

In college, I reconnected with Pamela. I was in nursing school, but I was unsure I was on the right path. "Can I come spend the summer with you on The Farm and see what midwifery is all about?" She said, "I will think about that, write me a letter."

I wrote her that letter. I told her I was serious and I would be willing to help her in her garden and make dinners. She agreed, and off I went to my old stomping ground on The Farm as a 20-year-old "midwifery assistant." With a smattering of beginner-level nursing knowledge, I fully expected to be an observer. Nothing happened for the first week, so I busied myself weeding her neglected summer garden and making dinner. One afternoon, she said, "Well, come with me, we have a mom who might be in labor." This was exciting and unexpected. We went to the home of a young single mother having her second baby. The baby's father was not involved, and her mother was watching her other small child, so I moved effortlessly into a labor support role. I did this instinctually by staying attuned to her every move, bringing water to her after a heavy contraction, helping her move positions, smiling at her, and encouraging her. She was so beautiful to me; she glowed. That night, all the remaining Farm midwives who still lived there made it to her home for the birth.

Though my mom went on to have four more children, this scene with Pamela was my first birth. Children raised on The Farm, for the most part, were expected to help care for their younger siblings, though they were also excluded from coming to their births. We lived communally, so several families and all the children would share a big house with parents having their rooms and kids often bunking together. When a person entered labor, the adults shipped the kids out to other households for several days. While I now know the value of creating sacred spaces for birthing people, what that meant for me as a young girl was I had a tremendous amount of responsibility caring for my siblings, but was not allowed to stay with my mother when she was in labor. Up until that point in my life, I'd never attended or even seen a birth.

So here I was as a young, wide-eyed apprentice, not far from the very spot I was born, watching a baby's head crown in the home of a young mother for the first time. He came out limp and pale, not crying. A "hard start," just like me. The midwives moved swiftly to help him breathe; no one said anything to each other; their hands knew what to do. About one in 10 babies needs help breathing at birth. Their little lung sacs are closed up in the aqueous womb, so when they are born and experience atmospheric pressure, those sacs must press the fluid out of the way, open up, and exchange air for the first time. With the cord still pumping oxygen-rich blood from their mother's placenta, and their beautiful little lungs trying to inflate, they "transition" to life.

The mother looked at me, "Why is he not crying?" I was stunned at the sight of the limp, pale boy and just stared back at her; no words left my mouth. I hadn't studied and learned about fetal circulation yet; I felt her fear. While the midwives were focused and hard at work with the baby, I remember watching his mother reach down between her legs and, grabbing his little foot, said, "Wake up, baby, wake up!" At his mother's touch and voice, his whole body startled, arms and legs suddenly muscular and moving. He made a cry, and I watched as the center of his chest turned the most perfect, beautiful pink. She picked him up and held him. I stared in awe, and reverence seeped through me with this moment of intimacy between the mother, baby, and midwives.

When I finally returned to my little loft above Pamela's dining room table in the dark early morning hours, my head was pounding and my body was exhausted. Still, I was absolutely certain this was the only thing I wanted to do with my life. Later that morning, I climbed down the loft ladder and joined Pamela at the kitchen table. She was slowly eating cereal and milk. I didn't say anything; I just sat in awe of her presence and my newfound heart's desire. "You're a midwife," she said. "You don't have all the information yet, but you'll learn it. You're a midwife."

This birth, this declaration from Pamela, this life moment set me on a journey to finish nursing school, get my master's in nurse midwifery, and ultimately my doctorate. I knew I didn't want to go the route of Certified Professional Midwifery, which would have meant only out-of-hospital births, but instead chose advanced practice nursing to broaden my career options. Pamela blessed this idea, and she told me I would be a "bridge-builder" to help hospitals understand how birth works. This blessing from her meant everything to me as I so respected the many training paths to becoming a midwife; they are all valuable. My career bloomed from birth centers into a busy faculty practice within an academic medical center, and currently, to integrated women's healthcare startups trying to reimagine how we care for women and children.

My midwifery education gave me the clinical foundation, but my true teachers were the women and families I served. Every birth, every shift, every conversation shaped my mind and heart. I tirelessly worked through days and nights, sitting with people in the clinics and birth rooms, listening to their fears, needs, wants, complaints, joys, and sorrows. I have lost more hours of sleep than I ever care to count, carefully tending to families in labor through the night, soaked in gratitude and awe.

I have had four children born into the loving hands of friends and colleagues. It was a chance to become the birthing mother myself, on the other side of receiving incredible care. I learned lessons from those births that impacted how I live, love, and approach my clients.

My midwife life is a treasure of experiences and understanding about the human journey.

Thank you for the invitation to allow my story to weave into the origins of your story.

### ORIGIN STORIES

Wherever you are reading this, whatever you are thinking about yourself, your fertility, your pregnancy, or your birth, I want to shatter something important: There is no perfect pregnancy, no perfect birth, no perfect parent. But with the shattering of perfection comes a rebuilding of a new truth: There is no more vulnerable time in life than the transformational space of conception, pregnancy, birth, and parenting. You are not who you once were, and you are not yet who you will become.

Here is something true: You are stronger than you believe, more capable than you know, and more powerful when you share your journey in community.

And here is something else that is true: This book reflects my lived experience as a white cis woman, midwife, and mother of four raised in a family-oriented hippie community where pregnancy and birth were front and center as a shared priority. I recognize that my upbringing is not representative of many women's experiences in their community or with their healthcare providers.

### SHARED CHALLENGES, SHARED STRENGTH

As we talk about community and origin stories, I want to speak directly and clearly about the significant challenges facing pregnant and birthing Black women in our health system. We know this is true because of the stories we hear from Black women and the significant volume of health data that supports it. In the United States, Black women are three to four times more likely to die in childbirth than white women[5]. That's not because of education or income; it's because of systemic racism and implicit bias in healthcare. Our healthcare system does not hold all bodies safely.

Despite spending more money than any other country on maternity care, we are losing mothers at incomprehensible rates. There is a wealth of information documenting how marginalized communities are poorly treated in our healthcare systems. Every birthing person deserves a beautiful, supported, transformational experience. When possible, Black women deserve to be cared for by Black healthcare providers who understand their lived experience. When that is not consistently available, Black women and their families deserve care providers who "interrogate structural racism and

[5] Centers for Disease Control and Prevention. (2023). *Maternal mortality rates: 2023.* https://www.cdc.gov/nchs/data/hestat/maternal-mortality/2023/maternal-mortality-rates-2023.htm

its resulting power imbalances ... and engage in actions that disrupt the status quo."[6]

There are incredible professionals at the cutting edge of advocacy, research, and education who are helping turn the tide on the staggering statistics facing Black women and families. As a white woman, I seek to be a supportive ally and advocate, continually educating (and re-educating) myself as a practitioner on ways to serve and build better systems of care.

I would also be remiss not to mention those on this journey in the LGBTQ+ community; the blatant discrimination and invisibility have also led to significant trauma and inequities. You are not safe in systems that don't see you and respect your choices, and this must change.

I share these origin stories and perspectives because I want to be clear: Some readers may find my tone and approach in this book to be gentle. For me, that gentleness is my own gift and strength. This gift has shaped my approach to care and informed my work in clinical leadership. However, I also hold a deep commitment to truth, and the reality is that birth does not unfold equally for everyone. There is room for all kinds of voices as we try to move forward in our conversation about improving birth culture together. I hope that any woman reading this can glean insights that transcend our differences and gain a new perspective to help her navigate her own pregnancy journey.

---

[6] American Medical Association. (2024). *AMA Journal of Ethics, 26*(1), E72-E83.

If this book invites you toward presence, let that presence include the courage to see who is left out and to join the mission to build something better. While I can't speak to everyone's experience with this book, I do know that self-awareness can move us closer to healing. Closer to breaking down systems that aren't working. And closer to replacing them with new ways of being.

I'll use the words "you" and "your," but if you're a partner of some kind reading this book, this advice is for you as well. If I use gendered pronouns for women, that's not meant to disregard the experience of pregnancy for trans and nonbinary people. So no matter who you are reading this, know that I wish I could meet each one of you exactly where you are and tell you how loved and brave you are. I'll do my best to say it repeatedly in these pages.

There is a birth and parenting journey ahead for you, made stronger in its connection with a loving community, sentient care systems, and the rites of presence. Presence is the place where we draw from the well of what is true inside ourselves. May this collection of wisdom, nurturing, and story connect and root you to your true self. May you learn to trust yourself and receive dignified support. May you find what you need on your way to this beautiful becoming.

YOU ARE NOT BROKEN.

THE HUMAN BLUEPRINT IS BEAUTIFUL.

# beginnings

*"Sometimes it's not about knowing the answer, but being inside of the question together."*

*– Andrea Gibson*

**WE DON'T** take teen girls to the emergency room because they found blood on their underwear. We give them a box of pads and a hug (hopefully). Some young women are met with a book and an awkward conversation with their parents. If you are a daughter of progressive parents, you might get a party or a ceremony. But for most of us, we're told through actions or words that we are now in a new phase of life, one anticipated, one that should be marked and celebrated as a rite of passage.

We don't pathologize the beginning of our fertility journey; we help each young woman embrace it with support. We have an opportunity to do the same thing with the next phases of our journey.

## BECOMING PREGNANT

The reproductive journey often starts, of course, with getting pregnant. This isn't a book about *getting* pregnant, though it'd be a disservice to cruise right on by that critical moment because it is the set and setting for your birth journey. And what a range of origin stories there are, dear readers. Ages that range from very young to very old, and timing from the very planned to the very surprising. Some pregnancies start after gut-wrenching years of trying to conceive. Some women get pregnant while using IUDs. Some are partnered, some aren't. Some partners are helpful on the journey, some aren't.

You may be reading this while walking alongside a surrogate who is carrying the cherished child you have desperately wanted. You may be reading it with the intention of choosing adoption. You may be reading it because you had a horrible birth experience with your first child, and with subsequent children, you want to do it differently.

The diverse experiences of arriving into expectancy will soon merge into the familiar rhythms of remembering, rooting, releasing, and receiving as the journey unfolds. This reminds us all that despite our different paths to this place, welcoming new life is a shared human experience.

## THE HUMAN BLUEPRINT

By now, I've mentioned the human blueprint quite a bit. So let's make sure we have a clear understanding of what I am describing. In molecular biology, the "human blueprint" refers to our DNA — the complete set of instructions that dictate human development. You may also hear some healthcare providers refer to the human blueprint as the health and intelligence inherent in all of us: the body's innate capacity to function, grow, and heal.

The human blueprint is the conductor of the natural hormonal orchestration during this physiologic process, directing hormones like oxytocin, endorphins, adrenaline, and prolactin to work together synergistically, as a perfect symphony.

For our purposes in this book, the *intelligence* inherent in the human blueprint is this hormonal cascade that mediates the entire process of conception, pregnancy, labor, birth, bonding, and breastfeeding. Oxytocin, chief among the neuropeptides in this cascade, is released from the brain and governs much of what unfolds during these stages, fueling contractions, bonding, and milk production. Levels of oxytocin peak as the baby's head begins to crown, leading to the powerful contractions that bring your baby into your arms.[7]

Each human body has a sophisticated nervous system mediating these hormonal processes and geared to help us protect ourselves along the way. Incoming stimuli — whether real or perceived, good or bad — can activate our nervous system and profoundly impact our experience of being human. Thanks to the groundbreaking work of Bessel van der Kolk's T*he Body Keeps the Score*, we have the science to understand

[7] Uvnäs-Moberg, K., Ekström-Bergström, A., Berg, M., & et al. (2019). Maternal plasma levels of oxytocin during physiological childbirth: A systematic review with implications for uterine contractions and central actions of oxytocin. BMC Pregnancy and Childbirth, 19, 285.

the relationship between our body and our emotional states.[8] Van der Kolk, an early pioneer in the study of trauma and the brain, emphasizes that emotional states affect our physiology. Stress hormones like cortisol aren't inherently bad — in fact, they serve a vital purpose for most of human history in helping us respond to threats. But their timing is everything.

While your acute stress response can activate your body to avoid a harmful event, chronic stress is marked by a continuous release of cortisol and other hormones throughout your day that can degrade your immune system and contribute to harmful chronic conditions. In labor, this stress response can shut down oxytocin and stall or disrupt the natural rhythm of labor, interfering with the reproductive hormones designed to carry us through. Van der Kolk goes on to explain that after experiencing a stressor, it is in *social connection* that we calm our bodies and come back into balance, allowing the human blueprint to continue its mission of balance and well-being. The young midwives on The Farm didn't have MRIs to understand why their care approach worked so well, but we do now, and it is a powerful clue to how we survived as a species.

## FACING FEARS, CULTIVATING CONFIDENCE

No matter how you got here, you've arrived. You're pregnant. You've crossed the threshold into a transformative journey. Along with excitement and anticipation, fear can emerge. Fear about pregnancy and childbirth can come through different

---

[8] Van der Kolk, B. A. (2014). *The body keeps the score: Brain, mind, and body in the healing of trauma*. Viking.

sources, both external and intrinsic. Over time, I observed that talking about and "unwinding" fearful ideas around pregnancy and childbirth with my clients took up large portions of the prenatal visits. Media sources play a significant role in shaping beliefs and ideas. Some of the most popular pregnancy books are page after page of warnings and sound bites for "what to watch for" and "when to call your provider." While we need access to information to stay healthy, many of us do not need more anxiety about what could be looming ahead. The United States is particularly guilty of this media bias and perpetuation of negativity. Stories that make headlines are often sensationalized.

If this is all you know about birth, it could become a negative influence. Just like you trust a trained flight crew to get you to your destination, vigilantly monitoring all signs and trained to handle all scenarios, healthcare providers, and especially midwives, are vigilantly watching for all the signs that a birth might be moving toward risk. It's not your job as a pregnant person or loving support person to absorb every what-if and worry. That is what a good team will carry for you.

So much of what we see and hear about birth is the very representation of disempowerment. This perspective of birth is not helpful at best and destructive at worst, especially when it triggers a stress response. All of these influences can obscure our trust in the intelligence of the human blueprint and disrupt the hormonal feedback loops designed to help the process work.

Thousands of babies are born every day, but you just don't hear about what goes right. Cultural fear around birth and pregnancy is not itself new, but the modern depiction in the media has amplified its impact. Pregnancy and birth have always been something to respect and hold sacred, but what we get exposed to now is out of balance: "Normal birth" is underrepresented, and dramatic scenarios with rare and often life-threatening complications are the media norm.

Combine this with the barrage of negative birth ideas promoted in film and television, and you suddenly realize you are in an uphill battle with culture and care models. And this misrepresentation has given us a limited imagination of pregnancy and childbirth. When I talk to people about my work, I often ask them this question: "Imagine a woman in labor. What is the first image that comes to you?" I almost always hear variations on the same theme: hospital room, blue gown, medical equipment, bright lights, and yelling.

How do we face our fears, calm our bodies, and trust our human blueprint? How can we begin to understand the effects of stored trauma in the body on our journey? This is a wide and deep topic because our human journeys are all unique, and what we may need to answer this question is diverse. Intrinsic sources of anxiety come from our own life events and exposures; they are unique to you. It depends on how you grew up, where you lived, your skin color, and so much more. Both major and minor life traumas can affect how we feel and think about pregnancy, birth, and parenting. For Black women, the evidence clearly indicates that the experiences of racism and trauma (both personal and intergenerational) play a significant role in shaping pregnancy and birth outcomes.

For all women, access to trauma-informed care is crucial for ensuring better maternal health outcomes. As you face your fears and seek to understand the source, choose healthcare systems that offer empowering trauma-informed care, and find a safe community for the journey. This is the beginning of being present for yourself.

There are also cultural fears. Our medical system battles structural racism that mistreats people of color across all disciplines. Studying why this happens helps us, as healthcare providers, acknowledge our own biases and take action to dismantle and interrupt systemic inequalities. The burden of change should be on the healthcare community, not on you throughout your pregnancy. Finding a healthcare provider who acknowledges this is an essential early step.

As we enter into our fertility and pregnancy journey, it is important to name this cultural, medical, and psychological phenomenon and understand its roots, one where fear, harsh realities, disempowerment, and lack of agency may shape the pregnancy experience. The information and stories shared here aim to educate and empower you to distinguish between real and conditioned fear. Our goal is to move away from cataloging all fears and instead cultivate a sense of confidence. So let's take a moment to look fear straight in the eyes, but with me staying present for you.

As a midwife, I have absolutely seen hard outcomes. But most of the births I've attended have been safe, joyful, and empowering. So let's start with the fact that fear makes imprints through our stories. Even among friends, it's often the stories of bad experiences that are more socially acceptable to be shared. I had a friend tell me a familiar tale of going to a dinner with girlfriends, only to overhear a new mom tell a pregnant mom her horrible birth story. The new mom went on and on, the story getting worse at every turn, completely oblivious to the fear it was causing the pregnant mom. My friend didn't want to halt the story and try to shame the new mom about sharing, so she kept quiet. But what she did the next day was to reach out to her pregnant friend, acknowledge the stressful experience of hearing that story, and share her own empowered birth story. This story illustrates how fear around birth can be so easily perpetuated, and how we need to actively make space for a new, more positive narrative.

I have had the privilege of caring for women from diverse cultural backgrounds and have seen the power of cultural connection and confidence around birth. The sense of awe and presence in these connected moments was familiar to me because of my roots in the commune.

Traditional cultures, those before modern medicine or those outside our American paradigm of hospital birth, were (and still are) connected to the cycles of life and the human blueprint, providing a much better path toward an empowered birth. Midwives stayed with women through labor, knowledge was passed down, and birth and postpartum care occurred within community. People living in community with each other experienced a balanced representation of normal birth and occasional complications. This was certainly true for me as a young girl growing up on The Farm. It never even occurred to me to be fearful about birth; it was part of our lived experience within the commune.

This can be your truth, too, even in our modern birth environments. As I tell you with every fiber of my being, I want you to know there's a better way forward.

### EMPOWERED BIRTH: A NEW PARADIGM

This new path forward is an empowered birth. This is defined as a birth that allows you to know and validate your birthing environment before you arrive in labor, choose your care providers and get to know them over time, and come with a set of intentions and a team of trusted loved ones and caregivers to help you build your birthing nest. The "nest" is the sensory environment that brings you easily into calm, into breath, and into presence and connection with yourself and your team.

Think of a birthing nest like a cozy little den that is your domain. It might be a thoughtfully arranged corner in a more traditional hospital room or the warm embrace of a dedicated space in a birthing center. This is what we mean by "rooting." Unless you're giving birth at home, chances are there's a buzz of activity happening around you isn't directly tied to your experience. Carving out a nest is a metaphor for ensuring wherever you deliver, it feels truly yours — safe, supported, and centered on you.

Start to think about your empowered birth not in terms of managing whatever you're handed, but rather as an opportunity to intentionally choose the safest, strongest, and most caring environment for you. That might be your home, a freestanding birth center, or a hospital. Make these decisions with the help of a trusted care provider who can give you the health information you need to know as you consider your options. I've been present at births in all of these places, and there is no right place to have a baby. The key to a positive experience is the family's comfort with their choice, a foundation of understanding about their health, and the ability to receive safe, respectful care that aligns with their needs. If you feel safest in a hospital, that is the right choice for you. If a birth center or your home is right, feel empowered to claim that path with confidence.

Your opportunity is to explore your reactions to all of the options. You must understand yourself well enough to know where you will be most at ease. Comfort created by the ideal *emotional environment* for you is the goal. The people on your support team, the place you choose to birth, and the power dynamics with your care providers make all the difference. If you want a birth environment that is, for whatever reason, out of reach, know you can bring the best elements of the nest philosophy wherever you land.

I came on shift one night at a hospital and assumed care of a mother who needed to be induced for a medical problem. She wanted to have the baby and avoid any issues, but she didn't love the idea of the induction. A few hours into it with the Pitocin going and an IV in her arm, she began to get agitated and said to me sharply, "All of this needs to go." She pointed to her IVs and monitors. "I want to take all this off and get a shower." At that point in labor, there was no reason why she couldn't take a break for a moment, so I carefully unplugged and disconnected her. She got into the shower, and her contractions kept coming. I sensed our nurse was a little sideways about this new plan, believing it would slow things down, but she was trying to be patient. We started to hear her moan low in the shower, and I asked her to tell me what she was feeling. "It's getting stronger," she said. Within minutes of this exchange, she was done with the shower and climbed back in bed in good, strong labor. She had the urge to bear down shortly after. As she held her baby in her arms, I had to step back and smile. I loved her spunk. She started with stress, but when she asked for what she needed, she was believed and listened to. This changed the story, and her body's hormones kicked in and took over. She felt safe and empowered, and her body opened up to give birth.

Here is what you need to know: *How you feel in your birth environment is directly related to how the process unfolds.* Most importantly, you need to feel seen and safe. You need to be with people and in a space that calms you down so the hormonal cascades have a chance to work. This is empowered birth; this is the setting for how the human blueprint inside you ideally unfolds. This is something every birthing person deserves.

### YOUR EXPERIENCE MATTERS.

When I ask my clients, "What do you want for your birth?" their answers often sweep aside the birth itself. "I just want my baby to be healthy," I would hear on repeat, as though I were a genie who could only grant them one wish. Of course, we want our children to be healthy and to enter this world with the best start possible. Here's the good news: Most babies arrive earthside healthy. You can hope for more than just a healthy baby. We've lost sight of how much our *experience* within our healthcare systems matters and what we have the right to expect from it. In fact, your experience is a vital part of your and your baby's health. How you are treated when giving birth impacts the very hormones you will be depending on for a successful labor, which is the human blueprint activating to work on your behalf.

As I cared for a mom in a routine prenatal visit during her last month of pregnancy at a birth center, I brought up the possibility of having to transfer to the hospital unexpectedly so we could talk through any questions she might have, which was a regular task all the midwives did to help families prepare for birth. "I am not going to the hospital," she said emphatically. I dug in a little deeper and told her the chances were good she would probably *not* need to transfer, but I explained talking through the possibility was something we found helpful for our moms. "But I'm not going, so I don't want to talk about this." I could feel the rising tension in the room as we batted these dueling perspectives a few more minutes. I knew something was energetically stuck here, so I redirected the conversation. "Let's switch gears and check on your baby, and I'll make sure we have an appointment together next week so we can circle back to this conversation."

When she walked in a week later, she said nothing and handed me a piece of paper with her previous birth experience carefully written out. She wanted me to read it. She had arrived excited and happy with her doula, only to be treated with disdain for wanting an unmedicated birth, gaslit by her care team, and totally unsupported in this environment. This was the traumatic experience that had cemented her resolve never to end up back at a hospital. With an appreciation of the hardship she had encountered and tears brimming in my eyes, I looked up at her and told her I was deeply sorry this happened to her. I told her a new truth as I pointed to her letter, "Even if you need to go to the hospital, *this birth* will never happen to you in our care. You have chosen a team that will treat you with dignity and respect, and you will be given options and support." She decided to believe me that day. By the end of the follow-up visit, we were both crying, and I gave her a big hug. Imagine my delight when she arrived in labor during one of my call shifts a few weeks later and had a beautiful birth. I can still see her in my mind's eye, sitting upright in the big bed at the birth center, nursing her newborn with a huge, permanent smile on her face.

I want you to know you are worthy of a beautiful, transformational experience. I want women to know their bodies — their human blueprint — was designed for this and they can ask for a personalized approach. Each person deserves a respectful, love-filled care environment.

## SOMETHING GAINED, SOMETHING LOST

When having a child moved from community-based births to hospitals in the 20th century, we gained some essential things, but we lost more.

We gained safer surgical techniques, assisted fertility, antibiotics, and better drugs to stop bleeding. We lost the art of labor support, the option to move around, eat food, and take time.

We lost the chance to hold our baby right away and give birth standing up, underwater, or on our hands and knees. We lost the option to tell someone to leave the room who didn't make us feel safe or whose own anxiety was mentally distracting us from the important task of labor and birth.

We lost community-based care and connection around the birthing family as they cared for their new little one at home. We lost reverence for the birth process, a sacred territory for transformation.

We have lost our connection to the important parts of the human blueprint.

But here's the fantastic news about the list of what we've gained and lost: They are not mutually exclusive. We can have it all. And I am here to tell you there are incredible hospitals, practices, and providers available to offer you the very best of modern medicine with a respectful care model that lets you be in the driver's seat of your care.

**CHANGE, BUT NOT FAST ENOUGH**

I have seen important changes from the late 1990s when I started practicing as a midwife. Some hospitals have positive trends around physical movement during labor, low intervention models, early skin-to-skin with your baby, and a focus on labor support from engaged partners, midwives, and doulas. There have been pockets of change, but we need more progress. And you have to know you can want it, you can seek it out, and your body was designed for this.

Our current birth outcomes in the U.S. tell the unfortunate story of too many birthing people not having access to progressive care models that support parents with loving kindness, shared decision-making, and a focus on supporting physiologic birth, a medical term that simply means *as our bodies were designed to do* when the focus is less on intervention and more on labor support. These progressive, sensitive models are the standard of care in many developed nations with the best birth outcomes, and need to be the standard of care for all women, everywhere.

### WANTING MORE

So when you are asked to think about what you want for your birth, and even if your baby's health is your first thought, now you know you have to take the answer further. These next chapters explore what you should look for in each stage of your pregnancy and labor journey to cultivate presence: tools for finding the right provider; how you should treat yourself; what you should expect of those who are supporting you on this journey; and foundational elements you want in place to nurture a positive pregnancy, labor, and birth experience.

It's OK to want more. It's OK to need things that may feel unique to you, that might even bring intimacy, laughter, or joy into the birth experience. Remember, this is a moment to be curious, to be educated, and to be self-reflective. It's your invitation to explore deeper parts of yourself because your and your baby's health is dependent on you actually acknowledging what your heart desires and what feels right for your birth. We can't control every outcome or detail, but we can tip the odds in your favor.

### YOU ARE ENOUGH

As we dive deeper together into what's possible for you in the magical moment of childbirth, I hope you will be able to fully answer, "What do you want for your birth?"

What kind of presence do you want to invite in? What are the moments along the way during pregnancy that will give you the clues you need to be in touch with your deepest desires for the birth itself? How do you need to be cared for, and what do you deserve to receive?

The world and culture around you may send you a faulty message that swirls around the idea of pregnancy and birth as a performance: performing femininity, the perfect pregnant body, the perfect labor and birth. Don't let this faulty thinking seep in, or even if it does, practice recognizing it and naming it as a false construct. You need to know you are enough, just the way you are.

This journey is about you, and it will take you into places you can't and don't need to imagine right now. Perfection is not the goal; presence is. Bring presence to yourself first, then to your body, and then to growing a human. You are first, you matter, and this is your life. You are not a bit player in someone else's movie. You get to decide how you will enter this journey.

You are the lead, and you are beautifully made for this time in your life. You are remembering and rooting in your power and intelligence, releasing fears, and receiving the support you deserve. You can connect with this intelligence through curiosity, self-acceptance, and community.

YOU ARE NOT BROKEN.
PREGNANCY IS NOT A PERFORMANCE.
THE HUMAN BLUEPRINT IS DESIGNED FOR THIS.

# first

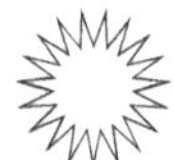

**IN MEETING WITH NEWLY PREGNANT PEOPLE,** I've trained myself to abandon the assumption this was a happy person waiting to start their prenatal care journey.

"Hello, my name is Margaret. I am one of the midwives. How are you feeling today?" With this blank canvas greeting, I sit and listen to the story of how this person exists in relation to the change they are experiencing. I've seen many different emotions in that first conversation: joy, grief, fear, ambivalence. Every story is unique because this is the beauty of being human.

As you begin this pregnancy journey, keep your mind and heart open. The diverse experiences and perspectives we bring deserve to be honored. There is no right way to do this; you get to start with a blank canvas.

**EMOTIONS**

We come to pregnancy by so many different routes. But why have so many of us allowed ourselves so few emotional options? We've all metabolized cultural narratives that we must either be ecstatic at the possibility of motherhood or upset because we didn't intend for it to happen. I say there is a wild complexity of emotions that is like Technicolor to this black-and-white thinking. So give yourself permission to feel your feelings, all of them, because early pregnancy is full of emotions.

When you're feeling them, remember to breathe. Be extremely kind to yourself. Talk about all of your emotions with someone you trust. It is OK not to be happy. It is OK to feel on the fence about it all. It's OK to have yearned to get pregnant or even sought fertility treatments, and then to feel scared it all worked. It is OK to feel like you want to return in time and not do this. You are normal; your feelings are shared by so many others who have journeyed this path.

We need to acknowledge joyfulness, as well as the full range of feelings and the infinite number of ways we digest this change. As you allow yourself to feel that range of emotions that will naturally flood in, you'll find that the people in your life who matter will be there for you in ways you never imagined. You just need to let them in.

When you let yourself feel all the feelings, it is easy to become overwhelmed. You are on a journey you can't always control. Not much in life is left in this category. We control literally everything around us all the time, so it feels weird and wonderful and terrible and thrilling to be on this journey. But you don't have to stay in that overwhelmed place. Like waves, let the feelings come in and then watch them go out. Recenter yourself on what you know and remember what is true about *who you are.* Use your breath. The pathway that connects you to that blueprint is *not out of your reach.* You've got this. You were made for this.

So be very gentle with yourself as the big emotions come through. Let your loved ones and community be there for you, and if you need more than what they can give, seek the support of a professional. Let them all hold you as you enter into this part of the journey. Being emotional isn't a weakness; it's authentic and valuable, connecting you back to yourself and preparing you for the journey of parenthood you are entering.

### CHOOSING A CARE PROVIDER

With those big feelings early in pregnancy, you also have some big decisions to make, and choosing the right provider to take care of you might be the most important thing you can do for yourself. This is where it starts: midwife or doctor, in or out of hospital? There are many practices that offer a range of paths, so if you're unsure what's right for you, look for an option where you get choices, and don't try to figure it out all at once. Most women don't start a pregnancy knowing what kind of birth they are looking for, and it is OK not to have all the answers in the beginning.

What you really want at that first visit is connection and someone who will take the time to get to know you. Should you be seen right away? Yes. There are strong benefits to you if you are seen early, mainly because this means you have someone to reach out to with your questions. And that means everything. It is someone who can be present to your needs, calm anxiety, and help you get grounded amidst rapid body changes.

Your instincts matter when it comes to the people taking care of you. The National Center for PTSD reports half of women in the U.S. will have experienced one traumatic event in their life, and 1 in 4 women experience sexual assault.[9] If you have been negatively impacted by trauma and/or sexual violence, the care providers you choose for an intimate life event are critically important. If it doesn't feel right, trust yourself. Transferring providers is common, and it's something you might need to do. You owe *no one* a reason for transferring; it's your experience, and you can decide who will care for you.

#### MISCARRIAGES

If you see spotting or blood in the early days of your pregnancy, take a deep breath and say, "I will be OK." Because it will be and you will be, no matter what unfolds. *And it's also OK to not be OK in those early moments.*

Spotting in the first trimester can happen, and many pregnancies progress on a totally normal timeline with no other significant issues. And, naturally, spotting can be indicative of other outcomes. Breathe. Reach out to your trusted support systems. Remind yourself, "I will be OK." Even if *this* isn't going to be OK.

---

[9] U.S. Department of Veterans Affairs. (n.d.). *PTSD research on women.* https://www.ptsd.va.gov/professional/treat/specific/ptsd_research_women.asp

Miscarriages happen. Maybe it was cells that weren't dividing just so, the DNA sequences inside the cells that weren't in the right order, or forces of the universe beyond our comprehension. The hard truth is that, for the most part, miscarriage is not well understood or explainable all of the time. Even the word "mis-carriage" is a tragedy, blaming the "carrier," as if you have ANY control over this spontaneous and common life event. A staggering 1 in 4 pregnancies ends like this. I am encouraged by a new movement to bring compassionate attention to pregnancy loss, reinventing the very word into "ThisCarried."

You are not alone, you are not to blame. Remember you are in the company of many women who have shared your experience. Please receive this message: Miscarriages happen, and it is not your fault. It is normal and common for women to comb through their actions and activities to create a link of understanding, to unlock a "why." I have sat with so many people, trying to help them hold space for the mystery of it and avoid self-flagellation. Trying to understand the *why* is part of being human.

A note about miscarriages and fear: At the time of writing this book, I would be remiss to gloss over the fact that in a post-Roe world, miscarriages and ectopic pregnancies have become a very charged part of political discourse, bringing with them stories of very real, tragic outcomes. These stories are not exaggerated, but the probability of something similar happening to you is low. That doesn't mean we don't take these stories seriously. They are an important part of our cultural conversations, and doctors and obstetric providers need to be trusted to make decisions that put the mother's health at the forefront of medical decision-making. But for you, in a moment of early spotting or unknowns, remind yourself that holding on to fears too tightly can compound the stress you already might be feeling. Return to your breath and your mantra, "I will be OK." And trust that the human blueprint, even in these kinds of difficult moments, is also designed to work in tandem with your body when a pregnancy is no longer viable.

You will be OK, and again, *it's OK to not be OK until you are OK,* so take the time you need to process. Seek loving care providers and clear a space in your life to move through this with your tribe. Take the time you need to collect yourself. Losing a baby on my own journey was the hardest thing I had ever endured, and it was the most transformational.

### TIME

In those early prenatal appointments, the first order of business is usually orienting to time. The clock on nine months starts from your last period, so there is an immediate confrontation with time. We measure the baby's growth in weeks and days and give you a due date that can feel like a tattoo (but it's actually an educated guess). Your visits are plotted out at specific intervals with specific tests at specific times, making everything feel very precise.

This invites you to think about time: Where are you in this continuum? Do you feel like you have enough time? Do you feel out of control and need lots of urgent support? Is time moving too slowly, and are you ready to get on with it? Being present with yourself in the evolution of time is an early start to the transformational part of this journey and a beginning point to becoming present to your needs.

### A BEGINNER'S MIND

The secret of the first trimester is this: Rearrange your life each day around what makes you feel better and do that as long and as often as you need to until you feel better.

It is this simple and easy to remember.

Everything may feel upside down to you, but this part won't last forever. Here's your strategy: What do I need right now? There is no daily nutritional pattern, so relax! Eat what sounds good to you, avoid what doesn't. If you want to walk four miles one day and then lie on the couch another day, do that.

Your brain and body will tell you YES or NO loud and clear, and the answers change daily.

See each day with a beginner's mind. You are not who you were yesterday, and you are not yet who you will be tomorrow. Staying in the moment takes a lot of conscious effort, but it's a valuable practice you can come back to in the early days of caring for your newborn.

### FIND YOUR BREATH

Profound waves of insecurity and anxiety may rush through you unexpectedly. Want to know about a superpower? You have it with you all the time and can access it right now.

Sounds too good to be true, right? It's already been mentioned several times.

It's your breath.

Breathe in deeply through your nose and then exhale slowly, twice as slowly as you inhale.

Do it again. You are activating the "calm down" center of your autonomic nervous system, your parasympathetic response. If adrenaline and cortisol (sympathetic response during stress) are the gas pedal, breathing is the brakes. Breath informs your body (and your little growing human) everything is OK, your body is safe.

The vagus nerve, the chief operator of the parasympathetic system, starts in your brain and runs down through your body, with pathways to all your major organs. It regulates how we breathe, digest, and respond to our environments. Polyvagal Theory describes the circular relationship between your physiologic and emotional states at any moment.[10]

You already know this body wisdom, the difference between feeling relaxed and happy in a safe environment or nervous and jumpy in an unsafe environment. Our bodies remember what we have experienced. We subconsciously scan our environments to determine whether we are safe, which occurs beneath our rational thinking. We are in a feeling state first and then experience our thinking brain. Becoming aware of this primal vigilance, you can engage your body in calm with social connection, breath, and movement. Of the three,

---

[10] Porges, S. W. (2017). *The Pocket Guide to the Polyvagal Theory: The Transformative Power of Feeling Safe*. W. W. Norton & Company.

breath is the easiest and simplest to access, and you can engage this intelligent system anytime, anywhere. The more you use these tools to calm down and reclaim your power, the quicker your body responds.

Breath and breathing are threads that weave through the pregnancy and birth journey. The breath can reframe a moment and remind you that you can choose another thought direction, a physical clue to your body and mind to reroute energy. Taking those breaths "tones" the vagus nerve, which has a role in releasing oxytocin from your brain, the principal hormone for love, connection, and birth.

Think about the breath as the tool to roll out the plans of that human blueprint, reminding your body it has all the infrastructure it needs. Begin to spend time with your breath, however it feels comfortable. It is a tool you will hone and be nurtured by, and you will begin to uncover its powerful effect on your body.

#### BREATH: A DAILY PRACTICE

Don't wait to use this breath superpower only when you're upset. Cultivate a daily practice and make this a time to connect with your little human. Put your hand on your belly, straighten your spine nice and tall, and practice breathing through your nose, exhaling twice as slowly as you inhale. Practice this breathwork in the shower or bath, a wonderful daily self-care ritual. Or practice this before you go to bed at night.

Even for five minutes, and truly, even for one minute, you will naturally align the intelligence of your body and send loving connections to your little one. You will let that parasympathetic response calm your system and release oxytocin for you and your baby. And here's a magical little bonus for all this great, healthy, intentional breathwork you are cultivating: You'll come back to it in labor and parenting again and again. Take a breath.

### THE FIRST VISIT

When you meet your chosen provider for the first visit, make sure it's long so you have time to receive and enjoy it. This is the visit where *you* are interviewing the practice you think you might want to deliver with, not the other way around. Are you pushed through a cattle-herding process where you get weighed, prodded, and handed a bunch of papers to sign? Pay attention to how the process makes you feel.

Important in this first introduction is how a provider obtains your consent. I would be remiss not to acknowledge this has not been done well, especially for people of color. Consent done well ensures you understand the relevant information, know the purpose of the intervention, including the risks and benefits, and have time for your questions to be answered.[11] Consent is not something like, "I'm just going to do a vaginal exam now." Proper consent preserves your bodily autonomy and balances the power between your provider's proposed plan and you.

---

[11] American College of Obstetricians and Gynecologists. (2021). Informed consent and shared decision-making in obstetrics and gynecology. *ACOG Committee Opinion No. 807.*

You are vulnerable and need emotionally sensitive people to look you in the eyes and see you, to find out who you are, and to learn what you care about. Midwives can do this (or not), and obstetricians can do this (or not), so while my bias is toward midwives for the care of healthy pregnant people, it's less about the credentials and titles and more about how you are connecting with the person on this journey to care for you.

We have depersonalized healthcare, likely when Cartesian thinking emerged: I think, therefore I am. The notion that we are all about knowledge disconnects us from the power of instinct and intuition, which live in our bodies and respond in real time to our surroundings. We have the neuroscience to understand this beautiful brain of ours, stacked in three layers perched on top of our spine: First and closest to our spine is the reptilian brain controlling basic body functions like heart rate and breathing; the middle layer is our limbic brain controlling emotions; and at the top of our head is our neocortex, the thinking brain. All sensory inputs come up through the spine and the lower brain layers to the neocortex. Contrary to Cartesian ideas, our brains are not wired just to think. We *feel* first, and *then* think.

If you FEEL like you are **not** in the right place as you sit there with the provider, don't go back. Find a new provider; you have plenty of time. Interview them in advance if that is possible. If you are limited in your options where you live, try seeing another provider in the practice. Of course, pay attention to what they say, but also listen to what's inside you. How do you feel when you meet them? How do you feel after you leave the conversation? You'll know where you belong. So many women turn to trusted friends for referrals. That's an excellent way to cull down a list, but keep an open mind. Even if there's a friend who aligns with you on many parts of your life, your experience is just that: your experience. Pick the provider you feel is right for you right now.

For partners seeking presence when choosing a care provider, this meeting matters for you, too. Talk to your loved one about your experience and create a shared dialogue to ensure you feel safe together. Your loving connection is the primary source of strength, the thread through this journey, and being aligned with how both of you feel with your chosen provider matters.

#### SHARING THE NEWS

People ask when it's safe to tell people about their pregnancy. Hidden in this question is shame. If you tell them and something happens, would they show up for you in compassion or judgment? What if you told them and decided you didn't want to carry out a pregnancy or were choosing adoption, would they support you? Tell the people who will hold you in it all. You need and deserve the support.

#### TESTING

As you close the first trimester, you will be faced with your first big parenting decision: whether to check on the genetics of your baby. The current available test takes a bit of your blood and gets info about the baby's genes from DNA fragments in your blood. Pretty cool! The test itself can look at genetic information, and the accuracy for each abnormality is variable. Some people want to know everything, and some don't. Ask yourself this: What am I going to do with this information? Talk to your partner about how they feel. Exploring your thoughts and feelings together before testing will ground you for the information that comes.

Over the years, I have noticed two kinds of people: those who feel better with more information, and those who feel worse. If knowing there might be an issue will stress you out to no end, take note of that. If going through your whole pregnancy and not being able to prepare yourself for a baby who may have a genetic disorder stresses you out, take note of that. Talk this through with your people. These disorders are generally rare, but they can occur; therefore, if you decide not to take any action or pursue any tests, that's perfectly fine. If you want to test everything under the sun just to be sure, it's OK. Making this first parenting decision can be hard because it intersects with your emotions and cultural norms, expectations, and laws. You may feel exposed to judgment, and you may also be at odds with the people you love. You may be facing stark limitations on your options because of where you live. Take those slow, deep breaths and stay tuned to your body. Take the time you need to decide; feeling grounded in your decision is important.

### THE SENSES

Your relationship to your sensory world will change. Orient yourself toward curiosity instead of resistance. Your tastes, feelings, and sensations are bringing you into new relationships with your environment.

As your body builds a baby, your brain will begin to detect what is needed for the two of you to thrive. It will guide you toward the best things for you and away from the rest. Vegetarians may start eating hamburgers. Suddenly, your beloved morning coffee turns you off. Many healthy eaters may find themselves gagging at the thought of kale and reaching for a bag of starchy, salty potato chips. While the media depicts women craving things during pregnancy, I've seen an equal number of people who get intense food aversions during pregnancy.

Bringing curiosity and openness releases you from having to understand it all. This is the beginning of rooting yourself in body wisdom — listening and responding with sensitivity.

Knowing is not the prized possession on this journey; learning is.

### FIND YOUR TRUTH

Information will pour in from trusted people in your community and through the media. I would love to believe it's all nurturing and what you need, but just a glance at media or culture and you'll see right away that if it's about pregnancy or birth, it's likely negative and toxic. And I have seen the pendulum swing both ways in this toxicity. I've seen women ignore the advice of sound medical professionals giving science-based directives, and I have seen educated providers completely ignore moments that needed patience, intuition, and nurturing. Both situations are a detriment to positive outcomes.

Choose your influences carefully and thoughtfully. Look for sources that balance information and encouragement. Seeing a list of "Don'ts" and "Nos" will be less helpful than positive recommendations of what is good for you on this journey. The popular books that have fearful warnings on every page can wreak havoc on your central nervous system, especially if this is the only thing you are referencing for educational support.

The phone in your pocket with all your apps and search engines must be tamed and quieted. Some of those apps and articles are "paper tigers," designed with warnings and rules that, while created to be helpful, in large doses can cause cortisol spikes that are harmful to our health. Information isn't bad, but it needs to be balanced. Don't make internet searches the only source of education for your journey. This also applies to friends and family who have suddenly become obstetric experts and dole out advice and sometimes even admonishments. The well-meaning but fear-ridden publications and people in your life must be put in their place.

Please hear this: Feeling nervous or fearful about this new experience is part of the journey. It's not about ignoring fears or trying not to have them. It's about realizing you've internalized many of them already. You do not need a new, longer list of fears and opinions. *Fear dumping* is not good for you or your little one. Remember the story of the friend going on and on about her horrible experience? You can hold a space for her story, put your hands on your belly while someone shares, and say to yourself and your baby, "This is not *our* story." Find nurturing, supportive sources of inspiration and science-based information and know less media and fewer opinions may be precisely what you need. Partners can be incredible sources of strength in this daily task of editing your sources of stress; trust the people who know and love you, and let them assist you in this part of life.

Imagine stepping right over this negativity bias into a wide-open and creative space that is *all yours,* balanced with grounded information and support. You can create this new landscape and fill it with loving people, affirmations, creativity, calming breaths, and positive energy.

### REALLY REAL

The physical, emotional, and spiritual transformation that begins to occur is subtle and powerful. Like a signal going in and out, you will start having more "normal" days that you are not either totally nauseated or exhausted (or both). These good days will come unannounced and can be surrounded by harder ones, but they are your early light at the end of the first trimester tunnel and a harbinger (hopefully) of fewer hard days ahead.

When you have a good day, you want it to be your new forever, so when you get a hard day after that, it doesn't feel fair. Do not despair! Remember, this is a good sign your placenta is growing well, and the hormones that initially supported the baby's growth are starting to level out. As the placenta begins to do the bulk of the nutrient and oxygen exchange, you will feel better. With your new energy and momentum, practicing becoming present to your changing body can invite joy. Good things are coming, and this journey is getting really real.

YOU ARE NOT BROKEN.
YOUR BODY IS STRONG.
THE HUMAN BLUEPRINT IS BEAUTIFUL.

# second

**PERHAPS IT'S IN OUR DNA** to notice and comment on pregnant people, the simple marvel and fascination at new life in the making. Our body undergoes this rapid change at no other time in our lives. Your familiar human form will become a source of wonder literally overnight: new folds and curves, changing skin, and lush hair. Embrace it! In its infinite wisdom and laser focus to build a baby, your body lays down life-giving layers of vital tissue and fluids. These tissues are round, full, voluptuous, and integral to your baby's survival. Embrace the intelligence, resist comparison, and celebrate the diversity of shapes and sizes that nurture new life.

**SHAPE OF YOU**

Enjoy your body as it changes. Say really nice things to yourself every day; this can feel awkward at first, but it is powerful and it roots your new emerging identity. Do all you can to release untrue media ideals that can lead to perfectionism and comparison. Comparison is a thief of contentment. We live in a culture that promotes limited ideas of beauty. Although there are glimmers of change, this will likely affect your pregnancy journey.

Each person will experience these changes differently. Your clothes fit in the morning but maybe not by afternoon, forcing you to contend with a changing profile. For some, this is welcome and hilarious; for others, it can dredge up body image stress. If you are reading this and somehow managed to grow up unscathed by body image issues, congrats! There's at least one of you. For the majority, the in-between of the old form and the emergence of a new shape can create strong emotions. Take a breath, remember the only thing you can depend on in this process is change. Treat yourself like someone you love. Embrace those comments as compliments, even when poorly executed by well-meaning messengers awkwardly proclaiming something as mortifying as "You're huge!"

Your body is a *true marvel.* Welcome this beautiful part of the human blueprint. It's an invitation on the parenting journey to bring self-acceptance and love, a practice you may need to return to many times.

## NUTRITION

When you have those good days, consider nutrition and hydration more broadly. Taking good care of your body is a fundamental part of bringing presence. Pausing to realize your daily routines need to adjust keeps you in the right relationship with the incredible work your body is doing. You are probably entering a new territory where you can focus on getting the right intake without battling nausea. This is important because the micronutrients you had on board pre-pregnancy were getting you through the early months, and you'll want the foods you choose now to keep those nutrient stores topped off for you and your growing baby.

During my first pregnancy, I fainted at work in the second trimester due to low blood sugar, which was very embarrassing as a midwife who was "supposed to know these things," but it was an essential wake-up call to the power of nutrition. You are building a baby, one bite at a time. You are also eating for yourself, so your body has to do the work of routing nutrients beyond the baby. Remember the first trimester when we OK'ed whatever you wanted to eat? We were just trying to get you through morning sickness. By now, it's (hopefully) cleared up, and you can start focusing again on being a smidge more focused on healthy eating.

Here's what you need to know: The baby will take what they need first, with or without you. This means the nutritive value of food is essential so you stay nourished, too. The closer the food is grown to where you live, the more nutrients it will have. Different colors mean you are getting a wide variety of vitamins and nutrients. Taking vitamins is great, but getting them from your food is even better.

Focusing on your diet doesn't have to be stressful or expensive, but it should be something you prioritize, as it can make you feel really good. Engage your partner or friends on this one; they will want to be a part of nurturing this baby. It can be a lot of fun. An excited dad brought a new cookbook to a prenatal visit to get my approval. He was determined to upgrade his cooking for his partner, and I loved his enthusiasm. Pursuing nutrient-dense food is critical for both of you, but most of all, you!

### WATER

Water is everything. *Everything.*

As the hormones that build a placenta begin to stabilize, myriad forces that shaped your first few months on this journey may organize into a steadier pace. If you get a sneak peek at your little one now, you'll see arms and legs moving around in a sea of critical fluid that you made.

And this makes sense, as we are mostly water. By the time you give birth, your body will have almost doubled its blood volume, and your baby is floating in a pool of hydration you created.

Make water a keen focus: Drink it, float or swim in it, be near it for relaxation. It is a vital life force, and your relationship to it matters. Not all liquids are hydrating, and your hydration level has the power to pump you up or drag you down. Make sure what you are drinking is actually hydrating your body, and imagine yourself as a well-watered garden.

### SLEEP (AND NAPS)

In deep rest, we restore all of the functions of our body. When one becomes two (or more!), the rest is needed. It makes perfect sense. Your body is working on its regular schedule, as is your precious cargo. Getting good sleep means releasing your previous definitions and embracing the new goal: 8–10 solid hours minimum. As I gave this speech to a very driven, professional patient, she gasped and said, "Are you out of your ever-loving mind??"

Your life might have been used to late nights and early alarms, but for this period of time, you are energetically completing vital tasks, and sleep is the only way your body can rebuild and repair. Protect your sleep, go to bed when you're tired, and take guilt-free naps. This is your new normal, and you will be better off to embrace it, full stop. To those who think sleep is for mere mortals and you are too busy to stay in bed, your body will sound alarms you didn't know existed.

A young woman in her twenties saw me for her first pregnancy, and by the second trimester, after several visits together, I could see a change in her skin and dark circles under her eyes. "How are you feeling?" I asked. "Fine!" she said with her best cheerful voice. I kept going, "How are you sleeping?" I looked at her partner, and they nodded at me as if to silently nudge me to keep up this line of questioning. What unraveled was her difficult job with a demanding supervisor pushing her to travel and work long hours. She was devoted to her work and didn't want to disappoint her boss. I listened carefully and gently said, "You are building a baby, and you only have *this* time to do that well. Sleep is critical to your baby's growth and your health." Big tears started flowing down her cheeks. With love and support, we helped her come into presence, to see that holding her boundaries at work was more important than trying to keep up with what she used to be able to do. This is what rooting is all about: noticing yourself changing and asking for what you need. She moved beautifully into receiving the message and releasing herself from these unrealistic expectations.

You need sleep and rest; you are building a human from scratch. As you hold space and become present for yourself in this new life pattern, talk with your people about what you need to support a rest-filled lifestyle. You may have to adjust to new patterns, and the support of your community is vital in making this shift. The energy you create at rest is essential to support the work happening in your body. It's worth it, I promise.

### STAYING STRONG

While your body gears up to grow a human tucked inside your abdomen, the functionality of your immune system shifts. This leaves you immunocompromised for the duration of your pregnancy. You are more prone to getting sick, and it takes longer to recover. In your pre-pregnancy life, you may have felt impervious to illness and pretty bold in your body confidence to fight disease, but this shifts while you are growing a baby, and it's best to revisit your habits and beliefs.

Practically, don't hang out with anyone who is ill, and consider wearing a mask and/or practicing social distancing if you have to. People may want to BE with you, but remind them they can't cut corners and risk spreading illness. Think about how you would handle it if your baby were in your arms. Would you risk being around that sick person? Probably not, so protect yourself in the same way. Be bold, blame it on your provider if you need to, but stake out clear boundaries to keep your body healthy. Everything you can do to strengthen your immune system matters. Boundaries are part of holding space and being present for your needs.

### VIEWS

Clinically, at this stage of pregnancy, we have options to gather all sorts of baby images and information about the little beings growing inside of us during the middle months of pregnancy. You can find out a little or a lot. Some images are for health and growth screening, and some are fun keepsakes. An ultrasound itself is not always perfectly accurate, so by opening that door, certain views or images can lead to further imaging, creating a sense of anxiety or stress. If this is your journey and you are struggling, remember your breath can bring you back to a calm place.

Determining the baby's gender can be a fun suspense on the pregnancy journey. A small contingent of people want the surprise at the birth, but the vast majority want to know as soon as they can, and sharing the news with a partner and loved ones is a treasured milestone. I had a mom recount how they decided to have their ultrasound technician write the baby's gender down and put it in an envelope. They went to a special romantic dinner that night and opened it up right after ordering their food. Their original "Is it a boy or a girl?" giddy pondering turned into a silent meal once they found out the sex of the baby, a little girl. Suddenly, a flood of new questions had opened like a dam in both their minds, and neither could speak for the rest of the dinner, lost in their internal dialogue. For their second child, they opened the envelope at dessert to spend more time wondering if it was a boy or a girl instead of wondering about all the other details that come with knowing. I share because sometimes *not knowing* can be a much more joyful, dreamy place to be.

**PRACTICING PRESENCE**

The early surge of hormones in a new pregnancy can zap your energy and turn your world upside down, but coming into the middle phase of pregnancy, you can begin to feel your normal life force returning, and it's encouraging. Yes, you are still you, and you can enjoy the things you love. Your person is growing in their little nest, and you get to enjoy a boost in creativity.

During this time, create a space for relaxation, creativity, reflection, intimacy, and gratitude. These activities create positive changes in your mind, heart, and body that you and your baby benefit from. Stress is part of life, but this new frontier of your pregnancy is a place to begin to notice those stressors and create balance points that unwind you and bring you heart-to-heart with your little person and your loved ones. These heart-connected moments release a powerful cocktail of healing alchemy for both of your bodies.

Consider making energetic space for a new human to join your life. As a wedding is to marriage, so a birth is to parenting. Once the proposal or the positive pregnancy test happens, all lines of sight are on "the big day." Yet a few precious thoughts or plans are planted and tended to for the next decades ahead.

Your life will change, and while it is a welcome evolution, it is still a change, and it will bring natural pivot points. There are so many decisions that need to be made about setting up your life to have a new person live in it. The excitement and stress of determining the answers to those questions are essential. Making energetic space starts with engaging your imagination, thinking beyond birth, and considering how your life will change. Explore this landscape inside your mind and heart: Dream, write, create art, and share it with your loved ones. Just as you might start premarital counseling, explore what support you will need for your new life with a baby. For first-time parents, everything is new and a blank canvas, and for those of you welcoming a sibling, your mind will be combing over introducing this new person into your family unit.

If you are partnering in presence, this is a place to engage deeply in the dreaming; talking through the details makes them less scary and gives you both a chance to decide which directions and decisions make sense for your life. Think about taking time off, who will be doing routine chores and making meals, and who will be tending to keep life afloat. Decide together how you will handle visitors, parental leave, and pet duties. It may seem silly as you read this if you are having your first, but I promise it is valuable.

This part of the pregnancy journey is not often addressed within the healthcare visits, but I found it to be an enormous area of the "mental load" people face as they near birth. Pausing, breathing, and connecting with yourself and your support community allows you to ask the right questions, connect with solutions, and get the calming clarity you need before your birthing day. If you don't have a strong support system, this is a good time to find a nonprofit or community organization that may help fill in the gaps. It's OK to ask for help.

Your plan is yours, and it doesn't have to meet an arbitrary cultural standard. In other words, don't get so obsessed with finding the right car seat or paint color for the wall that it becomes a way to avoid the deeper work inside your heart and mind. This is such a beautiful time to be reflective and introspective, letting the significant shift into parenting be a time to cultivate your personal growth.

### CONNECTIONS

Feeling a human moving around in your body is indescribable. It's an awe-inspiring experience. With it comes a sense of responsibility and earnest desire to protect. It's primal. My midwife observation is that telling a pregnant woman not to worry is like telling her not to breathe. It just happens.

Experiencing nervous energy as your baby grows is a universally shared experience. You can't always wipe it away or move around it; sometimes you must be with it. Breathe with it. Sit with it. The awareness and vigilance to protect is part of your becoming; it's part of the parenting journey. You can feel it big and loud or soft and quiet, but you won't be able to turn it off. It is there to bring you into intelligent alignment with what you need and what your baby needs. Often, I've found fears have themes. You don't have lots and lots of little fears, you usually have one or two underlying fears that are at the crux of those worries. Is it about money, abandonment, lack of preparation, physical harm, or becoming a mother? Something else?

Anxious energy can be your teacher; it can reveal what you care about. When you know the key things you care about, you then become empowered to care for yourself and also ask for what you need. This is bringing presence and receiving. Choose the people and resources around you to support your efforts in finding the right balance on your journey. Some of us need more help than others, but all of it is part of the process.

As I sat with a woman nearing the birth of her first child, she confessed her birth planning was not going well. She kept glancing at her partner as she gathered her courage to tell me she did not want her mother-in-law in the room. She blurted it out like a confession; I could sense their tension, but it was ultimately her decision. "Of course, we will ensure she stays in the waiting room," I said. She had been carrying this fear, and I watched as her countenance lightened after the confession.

Connecting with truth and naming her stress, she got to let it go and feel the wrap-around support that comes with birth planning. I validated her decision, and the three of us discussed how important it is to create safe birthing spaces. These things seem small, but they can make huge differences.

Invite a new way to think about the stress in your pregnant life. Stress in the natural world can bring adaptation, a form of resilience. The goal is not to have *any stress,* but instead to ensure the physiologic and mental burdens are not degrading your health. Think about stress as a tincture. You need a little bit, but there is a tipping point of too much. What is it? Each person will be different, but you'll know by your rapid heart rate, short breath, or racing thoughts. These are your cues to bring your body into balance. Practice breathing, connect with your baby, and focus on what you are grateful for. Talk to your trusted partner, family, care provider, doula or friend, letting the pent-up stress release as you connect with someone who cares about you. Social connection calms our bodies. Do this as many times as you need to in a day. Your body and your baby will be better for it.

#### SWEETNESS

There is a sweetness to the middle of pregnancy. The days bring communion with your little person tumbling around, and as the momentum builds to the last months, there is a soft and joyful invitation to savor the journey. Many of us (and I know I am one) can't stay in a place of unbridled joy for very long.

Brené Brown calls this "foreboding joy."[12] It's where you can't stay in a joyful emotional state because you're conscious of a feeling that this will lead to something bad happening. Relax a little, this is a shared human experience — to be both joyful and apprehensive at its fleeting nature. Our brains are wired to be vigilant and tend toward an inherited negativity bias; this is what kept our species alive. Our nervous system can associate being joyful with vulnerability. For marginalized communities experiencing systemic oppression, historical trauma, and personal violence, the weight of vigilance can overshadow moments of joy, making it even more challenging to embrace happiness. Acknowledging these mixed feelings and their roots can bring awareness to our experiences. Celebrating joy and success can affirm your sense of self and foster hope and resilience in the face of adversity.

So if resisting joy is a pattern for you, notice it and remember all life's events are impermanent; we only have the moment we are in. Permit yourself to feel this joy, all of it. And if it's helpful, be overcome with tears of joy, or name all you are grateful for. Make a gratitude list. Stay in that joyful place as long as possible, even if it challenges you. That joy is filling your energy bank, and we have good science to back up the positive effects gratitude can have in our bodies.[13]

---

[12] Brown, B. (2010). *The gifts of imperfection: Let go of who you think you're supposed to be and embrace who you are.* Hazelden Publishing.

[13] Seligman, M. E. P., Steen, T. A., Park, N., & Peterson, C. (2005). Positive psychology progress: Empirical validation of interventions. *American Psychologist, 60*(5), 410-421.

Bringing presence to yourself is about being in each moment as it unfolds, the joyful ones as much as the hard ones. How much more joy is there than feeling your little person stretching their precious arms and legs inside your abdomen? These sweet moments are yours to keep forever. And take videos of that growing, tumbling belly. I can promise your toddler will ask you one day to watch them repeatedly.

Many women also experience a surge of creativity and industrious energy, rearranging their homes to welcome a new person, attending classes to learn what to expect, and receiving love and attention from excited family members. Siblings pat the tummy and "listen" for the baby. Pets draw near as they sense something changing in their beloved owner.

Take stock of everything you have learned about yourself so far, how you have brought presence and welcomed change. You are on your path to your beautiful becoming. Make time and space to enjoy it.

YOU ARE NOT BROKEN.
YOU WERE MADE FOR THIS.
THE HUMAN BLUEPRINT IS BEAUTIFUL.

# third

**ARRIVING IN THE FINAL MONTHS OF PREGNANCY** can feel like a minor miracle. All the energy you have put into physical and emotional change brings you into a new territory: fullness. The fullness is felt in the body with your amply bloomed uterus and also in your psyche as you near the threshold of labor. A threshold is defined as the point above which something is true. In this context, what is "true" is that this baby is reaching the point of full growth, a full realization of the dream you've been carrying. You're approaching a powerful transition, crossing a threshold into the in-between, mysterious, and transformative phase known as labor and birth. It's a liminal space. You're no longer in one state (pregnant) but not yet in the next (parenthood). It's sacred, full of uncertainty, and deeply meaningful.

Living in expectancy invites many feelings: excitement, fear, anxiety, eagerness, curiosity, sadness, joy, and so much more. Trying to manage the regular ups and downs of life, work, family, culture, and this narrowing time in expectancy is something to be acknowledged. The world around you may approach it with reductionist comments: "You must be so happy," or "Ready for baby?" "Awww, this is so exciting." If you find it agitating or triggering, it's OK. The world means well (usually), but you must create a sacred space for your feelings beyond platitudes. There is a "you" in this baby-focused anticipation, a person going through a massive transformation.

Simply put: Moms get lost in the "countdown to baby," and it can throw them off; there is no more critical time to be embodied than the weeks before you do the most challenging thing you've probably ever done. You can find a place to live with the expectancy, releasing cultural narratives while still being able to connect with yourself. It's possible to do this on your own, but it's much more enjoyable with other people on a similar path, which is why community-based childbirth classes can be so powerful.

Today's childbirth classes can be virtual or in person and cater to your specific needs. Do you have to go to a class? Of course not! There is more than one way to educate yourself, but good classes also provide a safe, supportive environment to make connections to your body, your support people, and your baby. Classes are also a place to begin to practice presence with the incorporation of mindfulness.[14]

---

[14] https://www.mindfulbirthing.org/about

### DREAM

As you nurture your life dreams beyond birth, create a personalized space to process your feelings. If you want to, invite the people closest to you into that space. Writing or creating pieces of art can help connect to your feelings. If that doesn't appeal to you, just try sitting in silence and noticing your breath.

The more you process and understand the origins of your thoughts, feelings, and dreams, the more adept you will be at noticing what you need and how to calm your body. When you have thoughts (good or bad), your brain seeks out more of that thing in your environment. This was an adaptation of our brain for survival, but in the modern world, it can be a real challenge. Feelings and thoughts hold weight and can shape our lived experiences. This has significant implications for labor and birth, and we will return to it.

Be very gentle with yourself as you nurture another human inside of you. What you focus on grows; stay positive.

### GRAVITY

You will have a new relationship with gravity, and a sense of humor is the best way to live inside your days. This is not gravity as in seriousness, but gravity as in trying to get out of a car. Your relationship with your body can get challenged as it changes shape on you seemingly overnight. This time is both exciting and wild. There is nothing in life to prepare you for *this* type of body transformation. With all of your body's energy knitting together a human, you feel the fullness of gravity on your flesh and bones. The way is through, and the goal is a balance between movement and rest.

Frustration may arise when you cannot do something that came easily and naturally to you before. Body autonomy is something we often take for granted. Bring that beginner's mind you learned in the beginning to everyday activities and tasks as you near birth. Is there a better way to do it? Can someone else do it? Go on, have that friend tie your shoe! It's a moment not of dependency or lack of strength. It's an opportunity to laugh and connect.

Do what feels good when it comes to sitting, standing, or any movement. Your old rules and patterns might not fit. Be willing to toss them out and try new things. You can even amuse yourself along the way. Daily activities can take on all types of hilarity in your changing form. Everything in this realm is temporary; make it fun. Dance! Your moves will never look better. If you need inspiration, watch Amy Poehler's SNL pregnant bar skit "I'm No Angel," a positive pregnancy image to remember!

If this is not your first pregnancy, you will be contending with an older sibling who will want to be in your lap or have you carry them. What lap? What hip to perch you on? This is funny and difficult at the same time. Cuddling and caring for the kid (or kids) in your life while nurturing the one in your body is quite the feat as the pregnancy comes into the final months. You will need extra time for everything you do with them, as well as lots of patience and humor. You are sharing your body and building a baby. That alone is enough, every day.

I asked a patient expecting her third baby how she was doing as she neared her birthing date. "Fine," she said. "My children think I am the greatest mom in the world because I just sit and play with them on the floor all day. It's the only thing I have energy for." I laughed out loud and admired this wise woman taking care of herself.

#### GROUNDING

Explore your emotions like you would a new city and regard them with respect. Get curious and take time to listen. You have never been more hormonal than you are right now. Hormones are chemical messengers. When growing a baby, these messengers are very busy tending to your body and your little one. You will feel the largeness and importance of your hormones. Let them do their work and keep yourself calm, curious, and nonjudgmental — the essence of being rooted in your true self.

Anger may surface, and so may a feeling of being impatient and easily overstimulated. You won't be a zen master your whole pregnancy, believe me. The invitation is to recognize the feeling, name it if you can, and acknowledge what you need in the moment. Maybe you need quiet, rest, or someone to apologize to you. The goal is to feel your feelings and also know how to get back to your balanced baseline. This is the heart of practicing presence.

Take time to walk barefoot in the grass or dirt. Rooting yourself to the Earth has emotional benefits and also physical ones. This is called grounding. And while more research needs to be done, early evidence suggests that it can reduce stress and improve sleep. I met a birth professional who knew I had trained with Pamela on The Farm. She told me she had attended a workshop there while carrying her second baby. She sought Pamela's guidance about getting ready for her upcoming birth, as she was pretty close to her due date. "Pamela told me to walk in the grass barefoot," she excitedly recounted. She did just that and went on to have a positive birth experience. Grounding is a good idea, and it's easy to do. All you need is a natural surface and a few minutes barefoot.

#### GOING THERE

I had a patient who had a history of fast labor and was very afraid of not making it to the birth center and delivering in her car. We talked about this at every visit, and I could sense her distress. Finally, after knowing we had built trust, I told her, "Let's go there. Let's talk through the real things that could happen if you delivered your baby in a car." She was willing to go there. We had a tangible, graphic conversation about how a car birth might unfold. I answered her questions, and I saw her thoughtfully filing away all of the information. I could see her body language soften. The "going there" with her mind released the anxiety in her body, and she didn't need to keep bringing it up at her visits. She delivered her baby a few short weeks later... *not* in her car but happily tucked in at the birth center.

As time shortens to the birthing day, you may have fears and anxieties creep up. This is expected; it is part of the journey work. Deep down, fears are often our desire to exert control.

What can arise, and how can I be prepared to control it? The short answer for you is you can't always control it. It's the first lesson to accept as you enter parenting. It's the first among many, many things you can't control. It is OK to sit with these messages and feelings so you can unearth the deeper wish. Talk to your people, talk to your healthcare providers. Voicing your anxiety can diminish its intensity and allow you to understand it from different angles. Not tending to its presence can have the opposite effect of causing it to loom over you. Remember just because something arrives as a thought does not make it true; it is just a thought. Welcome it in, evaluate it, talk about it with people you trust, and choose *what to let go of.*

#### RELEASE

As you approach labor, it's important to lean into relaxation and release. Releasing tension in your muscles and connective tissues will directly help the path of your baby. Actively relaxing your jaw, dropping your shoulders, slowing your breath, unclenching your hands, relaxing your thighs are the beginning points toward this helpful release.

You've done so much great work up to this point, aligning yourself with a healthy perspective and healthy thoughts. This is important because our feelings express themselves in our bodies. Tense muscles consume oxygen, diverting resources from your powerful uterus. Practicing surrender and release as you near labor strengthens your ability to access that power while in labor. The connective tissues of your body are all wonderfully integrated. Relaxed muscles optimize the work of the uterus, making each contraction more effective and bringing you closer to welcoming your little one. What a paradox: You become stronger as you let go. It is such a valuable skill in labor that can't be overstated.

Labor brings a rhythm of uterine contractions mediated by oxytocin. Learning to "actively relax" involves noticing tension in your body, bringing awareness, and then releasing that tension with breath. The goal is to let each contraction be the main event and receive all of your body's energetic resources. The Farm midwives called these contractions "rushes" and placed a significant focus on helping the birthing mother with active relaxation.

While many factors contributed to The Farm midwives' successful outcomes, this focus on releasing tension through active relaxation was a big one. Think about something like deep-tissue massage or a loved one squeezing your shoulders. The person might hold or push into a tight spot on your body. The initial instinct is to tense up, but after that initial oomph feeling, you stay with it — breathing, softening, relaxing into the pressure. The same kind of intentional practice is what makes this approach of active relaxation in birth so effective.

It's life's most beautiful contradiction: relaxing as things contract, relaxing as things feel most out of our control, trusting the process. This tension and release is an embodied version of what it means to be human. What a gift we get to feel so deeply during childbirth.

**PARTS**

You are a multitude of parts. Part of you may want this labor to happen, and part of you is unsure you want to go through it. Part of you may want this baby to get out of your body, and part of you likes how convenient it all is, caring for your baby easily in your womb. Part of you may wonder if you are going to be a good parent, or if your partner is going to be a good parent. Part of you may wonder if you will know how to feed and care for this tiny human coming to live at your house. Part of you may wonder if your toddler will be sweet to their sibling.

Welcome all of your parts. They are trying to take care of you and bring you something good (even if it doesn't feel that way on the surface). Remember, your thoughts are not all facts; they are thoughts. Sit with the *feelings* coming up and gently bring presence to yourself.

You are sharing a space that ALL new parents experience. This space of not knowing and self-doubt is the metamorphosis that leads you into conscious parenting[15] — completely awake, alert, and attentive to yourself and your child. I have sat with thousands of pregnant people during this part of the journey. You are not on an island by yourself. *You are sharing this moment with humankind.*

---

[15] *The term "conscious parenting" was popularized by Dr. Shefali Tsabary, whose work invites parents to see their children as mirrors for their own healing. While Presence focuses on the birth and postpartum journey, Dr. Shefali's framework has deeply influenced how many of us think about parenting as a path of personal transformation.*
*(See: Tsabary, Shefali. The Conscious Parent. Namaste Publishing, 2010.)*

As a mother neared the end of her second pregnancy, she told me she was holding fear and tension because this was a boy, and part of her wanted another girl. Her brother struggled with all kinds of issues growing up, and that was all she knew about brothers: stress and pain. She was grieving something from her past, but it was having a real impact on her pregnancy. I sat and listened, validating her feelings. I could see that in the process of telling her story, she was shedding some of her layers of fear and also began nurturing hope that her daughter might have a different "brother experience." This fear opened up a wound in her that needed healing: something she was holding on to and something that had nothing to do with her baby but everything to do with her childhood. But in naming it and talking through the fear, she began to let it go. I had the pleasure of staying in touch with this mom as her children grew up, and I saw how much she enjoyed having a daughter and a son who stayed connected with each other.

The last part of pregnancy is a very poignant time, and feelings will likely surface. Remember you don't have to figure everything out. You just have to let yourself have your feelings, recognize your parts, and release tension from your body. You are enough, just the way you are right now. These are the kind of feelings that will surface over and over once you bring a baby home and watch them grow into spunky, wild little toddlers. Being in touch with your feelings at the end of your pregnancy is a beautiful, quiet time to work through your emotions and transition into parenthood. So get in touch with these different parts of you, usher in presence as you seek to understand them, and gently release expectations and fears.

#### BIRTH PLAN

Our feelings about the intimacy of birth are rooted in our human journey and are as different as our fingerprints. Some of you will favor touch; others will desire space. Trust you will know what is right for you. Do not apologize for what you need. Prepare your birth team with specific information so you don't have to process every little detail. Your care team should have a decent understanding of your preferences in advance. Have a birth planning meeting or write it down, whatever you need to make it clear. Think back to everything you've learned about yourself on this journey. When you imagine yourself in this labor, rank what matters most. This will become the map to guide the efforts of your caregivers and a way for you to let the planning part of your mind go offline. This pre-birth planning will allow you to stay in your body during your birthing journey.

My favorite thing to do was read birth plans, not printed off the internet, but truly from the heart. One plan asked for quiet right after the birth so they could sing a special song to their baby. When we got to that moment, and as she began singing, I felt the tears fill my eyes. That moment mattered, and her planning created the space for it. How beautiful is that? Think about what you know you will love and what you don't really want to deal with, and then share this with your birth team. This part is all about you.

**IMAGINE**

Visualization is a powerful tool to engage your fears and anxieties as your birthing day nears. I recommend doing this visualization exercise outlined below around the time you move into the eighth month — close enough to your birth but still with enough time to process what comes up. The goal of this exercise is to enter your labor with mental flexibility and the capability to reframe your birth journey if needed. I have witnessed many birthing families suffer through trying to adjust to last-minute changes in the birth plan because they had only one idea of what they wanted to happen. It doesn't have to be this difficult. If you process the emotions for different birth stories and imagine yourself easily pivoting to different birth paths, you increase your resilience. This will allow you to access presence for yourself as the birth journey unfolds.

Please hear this: There is a big difference between a conscious visualization and randomly spinning or obsessing about something you do or don't want to happen. In this exercise, you will have a defined experience of beginning, middle, and end. Sit still and tall, take a few breaths, say hello to your little one, and begin to imagine your birthing day. You will visualize two different births.

Let's start with the type of birth you'd consider precisely what you want for yourself. Slip into a feeling of positivity and a dreamy flow state. Go through the whole event: feeling your labor come on at home, getting into the car, driving to your birthing facility (or the arrival of your birth team if it's a home birth). Visualize a dilation check, a heartbeat check, working through strong waves of sensation, pushing your baby out, bringing your baby skin to skin. Think of all the details and go through the whole labor, birth, and bonding in your mind.

Now let's picture the alternative scenario to that. Rather than being in a dreamy flow state right at the outset for this visualization, come to a place, perhaps, where you're a little more alert. Think about some birth scenarios you may dread. This will be different for different people, so it's important to unearth what is relevant to your story intentionally. Make a quick list of a few scenarios you don't want. We're not going to stay in this line of thinking for too long, but it's essential to know even if something goes in a direction you wouldn't wish for yourself, you can still meet your baby there with love and positivity, rather than fear.

Imagine this *unwanted* scenario and go through all the details. Hearing the news that you need to take a new route, talking to your healthcare providers about what options you have in the new scenario (things like being hospitalized for monitoring, or surgery, or induction, or whatever you didn't want), but picture how they will be resolved with expert care, love, and support. Find a mantra that works for you, "I'm safe, and this is what's best for the health of the baby," or "I'm safe, and what my baby needs is aligned with what I am capable of." And then, as the scenario starts to resolve in your visualization, slip back into the flow state again, imagining yourself welcoming your baby in your arms.

Where did your mind go? What images, feelings, beliefs, fears, or joys flooded you? Where did you feel this in your body? Journal about it, talk about it. The information that floods in will be related to your internal emotional landscape. It is a powerful teacher and, if respected and welcomed, can help you on the real day. Visualizing is an *emotional practice* for this transformative journey. It helps your sympathetic nervous system (fight, flight, or freeze) welcome this athletic, intense, exhilarating process. It helps prepare your parasympathetic nervous system (rest, digest, calm), ushering in a rhythmic acceptance of this opening your body will be doing. Labor and birth are not just something you achieve; they are something you receive.

Process what comes up for you in both birth scenarios with your loved ones. The imagination has a powerful effect on your ability to bring calming neurochemicals into your birth journey. If we anticipate something, we are more emotionally and physically grounded and prepared for it if it happens. There's a difference between entering a birth feeling empowered and entering a birth trying to exert control. Feeling grounded and prepared — empowered — means you will have less cortisol and a better parasympathetic (calm) response. This is the art and practice of bringing presence.

#### REFRAMING

The ultimate purpose of the visualizations is to strengthen your ability to *reframe.* Reframing is shifting your perception about a situation to give it new meaning, new clarity. Why is reframing in childbirth so valuable? Things can happen as a pregnancy nears birth. Your body may begin to experience internal stressors. Your baby can move into positions not compatible with being born vaginally. Your labor may be very fast or very slow. These variances have always been a part of the process, and before modern medicine, some of them could become life-threatening to the mother and child.

We now have interventions to solve these unexpected complications around birth, and your healthcare provider will help you expertly navigate through them. These events are often out of your control, but what is under your control is how you reframe what's happening and the story you tell yourself about it. Where you have lost "control," you can reframe the way you are *thinking about it.* This isn't about asking you to minimize or gloss over any pain or worry. Reframing is about giving yourself a well of strength to drink from. It's a new mantra, like "I have a great team who will help me navigate any challenge." Reframing changes your neurochemistry for the better.

A mother arrived at the hospital in labor, and I could tell by her trembling thighs she might be pretty far along in the process. After a gentle assessment, I let her know she was almost fully dilated and may be feeling the urge to bear down soon. "What?" she said incredulously. "I need more time, I want time to get ready...this is moving too fast." She needed a moment to grieve *not* doing all her planned labor activities, which sounds strange because so many people hope for a fast labor. But hers was too fast and didn't match her expectations. She got a little tearful, and I did my best to stay in the moment with her. "I wanted more time," she said again, and thoughtfully, I replied, "We have all the time there is. Close your eyes, take a big breath, and let's get ready to welcome your baby." She did this reframing beautifully, and her kiddo was born shortly thereafter.

Focus on the ***what is*** of the moment, not what you thought it to be. Breathe. Letting go of what you thought might happen and what your new options are requires you to reframe the journey. It is the breath that can cue this process of reframing and remind you that you can choose another thought direction, a physical clue to your body and mind to reroute energy. You imagined you would summit this path on a specific trail, and you were given a new route at the last minute. You are still going to the summit; you will give birth.

You practiced for this moment, so use what you learned in your visualizations. Allow yourself to have feelings about the change and take the time you need for this reframing. Hold on to a new mantra: "I am empowered as I open up to a new path."

When needing help or interventions, ask yourself: What do I need right now? What is most important to me on this new trail I didn't foresee? Talk to your birth team and your providers about what support you will welcome, and then take the time you need to visualize yourself on this new path. Many mothers have had to reroute; you are in good company. You will get there.

A strong mother, having her first baby, arrived at the birth center almost fully dilated. She had a sweet, joyful team, and as I helped her out of her underwear, I noticed something dark brown on her pad. "Hmmm," I thought. I gently checked her dilated cervix and traced the perfect contours of a baby's bottom. The baby was breech, with meconium (baby poop) to boot, which explained the pad. I gently removed my hand, let the next wave pass, and looked her deep into her eyes, "Your baby is not head down, so we will need to go together to the hospital."

About three percent of babies don't line up head down, but instead orient with feet, knees or butt first. When surgical birth became safer, the skill of delivering breech babies became a lost practice. If you face this situation on your journey, please know that the experience and skill of the person taking care of you in a breech birth matters. The Farm midwives and local doctors delivered many breech babies safely. You may or may not have the option to consider this type of birth; it will depend on the training of your caregivers and where you give birth.

For this mom, delivering by cesarean was the path forward. She started laughing to relieve her shock and stress, and we hugged for a minute. There were some tears. I talked her through the steps and stayed with her as we received care at the hospital. After she had her baby in her arms and we were all back together, we talked about how it unfolded and marveled at this perfect little person in our midst. She moved me with her trust, her acceptance, her humor, and her love. This is the power of reframing. That was her beautiful birth, even in its surprise ending.

Commit to the journey. Be willing to trade in that map for a new one, knowing that you will find your destination. Remember you were made for this, however the journey unfolds.

**THRESHOLD**

Giving birth is intimate. When you think about the vulnerability of entering your chosen care place and receiving help and interventions from a group of people you may or may not know, it may feel daunting, but you are prepared. You have been preparing for this threshold, and you will lean into your chosen, trusted support team you invited on this journey. They can help you settle in for this intimate event, and you can stay focused on your breath, your body, and your baby. Visualize yourself in the center of a heart-connected care team receiving love and support in your birth space. With love in your heart for your baby, love for your incredible body, and love in the room for you as you work through this journey, you will welcome your little one earthside with equal parts relief and wonder.

YOU ARE NOT BROKEN.
BIRTH IS NOT BROKEN.
THE HUMAN BLUEPRINT IS BEAUTIFUL.

# labor & birthing

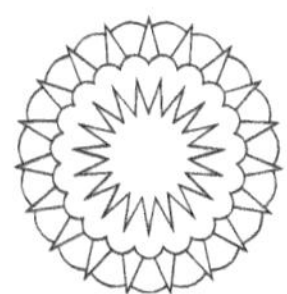

**WAITING FOR LABOR** is an ancient, timeless connection among all birthing mothers. Think back into the span of humankind: So many mothers heavy with child have sat and wondered when they would go into labor. The shift moves from the sweet feeling of waiting for a baby to the mildly torturous feeling of wanting to get something over with, like the last 10 minutes of a grueling workout, multiplied by nine months. "Can we just be done now?" might start playing on a loop for you. For those who have given birth before, it almost makes you giggle to remember your former, much larger self. You are sharing a space with these mothers, and the modern world has few moments like this left. We carefully plan the significant celebratory moments of our lives, so it is hard to wait and sit without knowing when it will begin.

Here is what we do know: There is a beautiful mystery around when labor starts. Theories abound, but it is not fully understood. In waiting, there is an opportunity to integrate all of your parts, and in that patience, parenting energy is formed. Children require ample amounts of patience. What if our time in waiting for labor was also our portal to becoming that patient parent?

And here's a little note on waiting: The more we manipulate a normal process, the higher the probability of needing more and more interventions. While there is a time and a place for a medical intervention to help start labor, those interventions should have a sound medical rationale behind them.

### TRUEST SELF

Labor opens a door for us to leave the territory of our "observed self." The self that says sorry, modulates our voice, and edits anything that could be conceived as socially inappropriate or offensive. In labor, you simply can't keep up that facade and truly enter into the sensations and needs of your body. You become the raw, unfiltered, and power-filled "true self." The truest version of you that may scream, grunt, fail to say sorry, strip off your clothes, and sometimes openly flail (this was me, for all four labors, and I added in ripping off my fetal monitor and throwing it across the room at the last one). You begin to dance with yourself in unimaginable ways as you enter the liminal space of labor; you are neither the pregnant person you were nor the parent you will become. You are your truest self, and it can be exhilarating. This has nothing to do with whether you choose medicated or unmedicated birth. It's true about all births.

This unfolding of the truest self is my favorite labor phase to witness. In our true self's raw, unfiltered arena, we access our authentic power, which is the rich territory of personal transformation. I remember a young, powerful mom doing beautifully as she worked through her first labor; I was impressed with her tenacity and patience. After several trips in and out of the shower, I got curious about her tattoo, which was written in another language. I took a minute to look up the translation: *She flies with her own wings.* She certainly did, embodied in her truest self.

You can be wild and powerful on purpose. Embrace this, you were made for it.

## BALANCE

Let's talk about "interventions" in labor, as this is a hot topic that inevitably comes up with birth planning. Accepting interventions was referenced when we discussed the process of reframing, so let's take a philosophical look at intervening in a "natural" process.

Many years ago, I stumbled on an economic concept called the Yerkes-Dodson law, which outlines the inverse relationship between intervention and outcomes. This is a principled explanation for the old adage "too much of a good thing is not good."

I had an epiphany about interventions in labor. I've spent my career caring for people across a vast continuum:

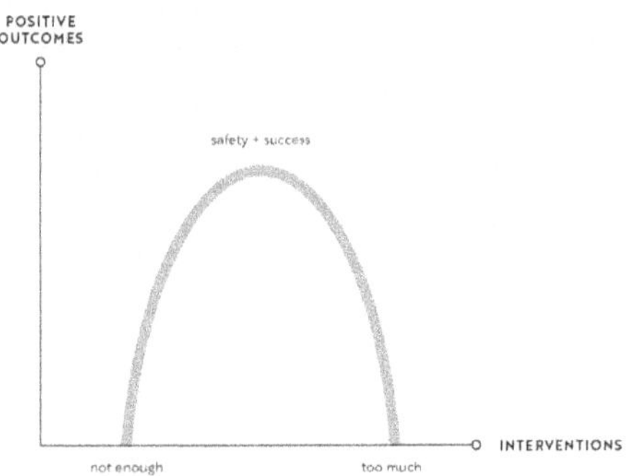


medicalization of a normal process

those who want no intervention and are willing to go to dangerous extremes avoiding help, to those who desperately need interventions and don't get it because they can't afford or access it, to those who accept intervention and have excellent outcomes, to those that intervene for no medical reason based on fear or convenience and have unwanted outcomes.

I applied the Yerkes-Dodson law with my midwifery lens, which fit perfectly. With no support, care, or interventions at all, poor maternal or neonatal outcomes are common. Good care with education, prenatal visits, labor support, and a loving approach, *even with medical interventions,* can create desirable outcomes. Too much intervention that bypasses the intelligence of the human blueprint can create the medicalization of a normal process and unwanted outcomes.

Why is this important? As you near the end of pregnancy and begin to think about your birth, please keep in mind the balance of action versus patience. What are the most important things happening right now? How can you support both yourself and your baby? What is your intuition telling you? How are you trusting the process? Stay present for yourself as you seek solutions with your healthcare provider and your community of support.

You know your body; you know you. You can have strong ideas of how you want your baby to be born. What you must hold gently is you won't know how your baby needs to be born until you are in the dance together. You did the work of visualizing and practicing reframing at the end of pregnancy, and this is where you might lean into using it.

Little ones can approach the birth journey in many different positions, sometimes making it difficult or even impossible to be born through the pelvis vaginally. Some have their hand over their head, or are not head down at all, or have a cord coming first — all of this making it necessary to rearrange the plan. Sometimes your placenta, the life-giving organ to the baby, sends signals of distress or blocks the entrance to the birth canal. Birth providers have ways of helping in these situations. These are your moments to get the information you need from your care team, connect with your baby, and consider accepting interventions. You are still the parent, and you will all be together on the other side, no matter how your baby needs to be born. This is what the parenting journey is all about: You show up with your plan, and your kid comes with their plan, and sometimes they are not the same!

If your plans change during the throes of birth, be ready to change too. You have prepared yourself to pivot if needed with visualizations and reframing. It's OK to slow down and get all your questions answered; that is a critical ingredient when a change of plans happens. It's OK to ask, "Do I have some time?" If it's an emergency and you don't have time, find a way to shift into the process of trust quickly. If you do have time, then it's OK to slow things down.

Sometimes, when slowing down, you will realize a decision is being pushed on you, and you are not ready, or this is not an actual emergency. Take the time you need, get the information, and breathe. Be prepared to be brave for the critical moment of reframing your birth path, or be brave enough to take the time you need to make that decision. You need time to see the shape of the story unfolding, see your place in it all, and find your footing. Not all interventions are suggested for your well-being; sometimes, there are system-based pressures, and it's hard to know what to do. Choosing a provider who has supported your birth plan all along, or bringing a doula or trained birth professional, can help you move through these moments.

You are capable of this transformation, and your little one needs you to stay present for the *what is* unfolding. I have sat with so many people in these difficult moments, and if it's helpful, I find the right moment to validate their effort: "This is hard, and this is the beginning of parenting."

**PRACTICING PRESENCE**

As a young midwife in training, I spent all day laboring with a mother who had prepared for natural childbirth and who wept when she realized she needed to get an epidural and Pitocin. I sat with her and comforted her as she grieved her plan that didn't work out. She finally had her baby, and as I was removing my gloves and washing my hands, the nurses said, "Margaret, there is a person who just got here and she is about to give birth, come quick!" When I entered the room, she was screaming for anesthesia to get her an epidural. She was almost fully dilated and nearing the birth of her second baby. I knew she was going to give birth before anyone from anesthesia made it to the room to begin prepping her back for an epidural. I was right, the baby came moments later, and as I sat with her in the aftermath, baby in her arms, I comforted her as she wept and grieved her plan that didn't work out.

These women wanted each other's birth plan that day, and the only thing that separated them was their expectations.

This is not just what I have seen happen; it is what I have personally experienced, too. I was humbled in my third labor when my labor got stuck and stopped making forward progress. A busy midwife and mom during those years, I was expecting this third labor to follow the same path as the other two: unmedicated, steady progress, and pushing the baby out. Nope. What I got was a stuck labor and a son who entered the birth canal at a funny angle (thus the slow progress).

This labor was longer than my first one, and when my energy became depleted and my stress and fear started to kick in, my contractions spaced out. After many attempts to get things on track, my midwife told me I needed to consider Pitocin. I told her I didn't want Pitocin without an epidural because I was physically and emotionally spent. She said, "OK, then let's do that." And so I did, and then promptly took a nap. In deep relaxation with anesthesia and with a bit of help from Pitocin, I fully dilated and pushed him out a few hours later. I learned firsthand (and very humbly) the power of pivoting and accepting help.

The birth you get may not be the one you planned, but it's the one you have.

### NEST

Birth works really well, most of the time. The environment created around your birth is paramount to the process. Let's talk more about how to make a safe place and create your perfect nest for this important time in your life.

The Farm midwives knew this truth about the environment of care. Remember my dad's fear about getting kicked out of his kid's birth? The midwives were clued in to the power of the environment and promoted a love-filled, movement-oriented, comfort-focused approach. They pulled the best parts of traditional midwifery knowledge into carefully curated, safe spaces for each family. None of these "spaces" were fancy, but they were comforting. What makes you feel comfortable is something you get to define and share with your birth team.

When our body senses tension, fear, or newness, it can react by clenching. This is often unconscious. Arriving in your birth space, meeting veritable strangers, and then being asked to change into a gown that exposes the backside of your body is the common scenario for many people going into labor. This is often counterproductive for a laboring person, and you can do it differently.

Get familiar with the route to the facility, where you will park, and the smell of the hall when you get off the elevator. Try to see the type of rooms you will be given in advance, how they are laid out, and how the light comes in through the windows. Engaging your senses in the birth space before you arrive in labor helps your body and mind "mentally map" it for your birthing day. We are generally more relaxed in a space that we are familiar with. If we feel before we think, it is essential to feel good in your birth space.

The best nest for you will be personalized based on your sensory preferences. The space you choose might already be precisely what you need with no help, but it could also be a blank canvas you need to customize. Bring in the elements that foster comfort and connection through your senses. Focus on what calms you down and brings joy.

An easy place to start is having preferred clothing, blankets, and pillows you love.

Your sense of smell becomes heightened in labor, so proactively bring something good (a candle, a blanket with a scent, or an aromatherapy diffuser). The part of our brain that processes smell is right next to the part of our brain that processes emotion. Smell is a powerful sensory cue that can calm you down. Take time to think through how you want your safe space to smell and what would be pleasing and calming to you.

Pack your favorite water, snacks, and other tasty treats. These delights can bring pleasure and an energy source. What your eyes rest on matters too. Among all the senses, humans prefer seeing the most. Many people bring pictures of pets, children, or ultrasound images to gaze at and feel connected. I've seen people hang up flags, post birth affirmations, and even bring in art objects. Seeing something we love or something that inspires us can be instantly grounding. I've also seen people take clocks off the wall or remove items from view. Editing the space is sometimes a vital intervention as well.

As we imagine the experience of labor and birth, music and sounds matter too. Playlists can bring energy and momentum. I love that people take this so seriously and curate birth playlists. I have heard some incredible music and seen its power to inspire, calm, and comfort. Music can connect us to our authentic, true selves. Enjoy your journey; choose sounds that bring you energy, peace, and joy. It could also be the case that you will need to block out distracting sounds, so having noise-cancellation options can also be a game-changer.

Building your birth nest might feel intimidating, but just look around your home, room, or favorite places. What are the elements that matter to you? What are your favorite sensory pleasures? If you are having a home birth, you still benefit from going through this nesting process. You may have all of your favorite comfort items close by, but you must be thoughtful about not being distracted in your familiar environment.

The dream for our future is that all birth spaces meet the basic safety and experience needs of each birthing person. Healthcare administrators, visionary entrepreneurs, and so many brave providers are trying to make this a reality, and the good news is hospital systems are recognizing the need and stepping up. However, there is still more work to do. Birth planning with your care providers is the first step in co-creating the right space for you. As best you can for your chosen birth destination, begin to weave your ideas together. As birds collect matter from their environment to make a nest, you can focus on this collection of details to optimize your birthing nest.

#### INVITING LABOR

Your labor will finally arrive. Welcome it and breathe. As each wave comes upon you, remember your breath is your body's reminder you *want* this laboring strength to build, you are welcoming this big energy, and you desire for your uterus to gently move your baby down the birth path and into your arms. Welcome your labor, greet it, breathe, and let it be as large and loud as it needs to. Let the love and presence you have created around you carry you through the journey.

I spent about three days in and out of early labor when I had my first baby. Being a midwife at the time, I was way too in my head about it all — writing down contractions, trying to figure out when the "real" labor would come. Tired and confused by day three, I called my midwife for a pep talk. "It sounds like you need to get into a warm shower and welcome your labor." Welcome my labor? What did she mean? Of course, I wanted to go into labor! But when I stripped down and stood in that warm shower, witnessing my full pregnant form and being present for my feelings, I realized I was very nervous and scared. And so I did what she told me, I took a deep breath and welcomed my labor. I said out loud it was OK if things needed to get stronger. I felt courage and strength build inside of myself. Early the next morning, I was holding her in my arms.

### BIG ENERGY

Labor is *big energy*. How it comes to you the first time will stay a mystery until you experience it. No one can tell you precisely what you will feel; they can try to describe different elements, but the actual journey will be yours and unique to you. Your body, in its intelligence, releases endorphins (natural painkillers) during labor, similar to what happens for long-distance athletes. Endorphins reduce uncomfortable sensations and bring a sense of well-being, sometimes even euphoria. The alchemy of the hormones released from your brain, the receptors in your uterus, these endorphins, and the neural pathways mix with your life history and your relationship to the sensory world, making your experience unique to you.

I have witnessed thousands of women in labor and seen dramatic differences in how they move and flow with their contractions. I have seen people entirely intolerant of even mild, early contractions, all the way to people who arrive for a routine prenatal visit complaining of "low back pain" and with a quick check were found to have a baby's head crowning, completely oblivious to their labor. These are dramatic examples and not the norm, but any midwife can attest it does happen. How is this explainable? We are all different, and our experience of this big energy is relative to our unique human journey. Your labor will be *yours.*

#### MAKE SOME NOISE

Be noisy. Why not? With big energy waves in labor, you will make sounds, and this is a powerful part of the opening your body is trying to do. You may never have roared, but you may need to do just that. Do not worry about how that will make other people feel (it's not about them, it's about *you*). You deserve to labor unedited by the people around you or the place you are in. Roar, moan, weep, scream, pant, grunt, cry out. These sounds are you, your truest self; they are your power and source of strength. Your baby feels the vibrational energy you make with your sounds, and it will help your little one on the birthing journey.

As a young nursing student on the maternity floor long before I had trained as a midwife, the instructor ushered us into a room of a patient who was "about to push." She lay quiet and still in her bed with her eyes closed. Coming from The Farm, I knew women giving birth made noises. I have vivid memories of hearing the strong moaning sounds coming through open windows of various houses on The Farm as women were laboring. The silence in this hospital room I was witnessing made me nervous and fearful. "Oh no," I thought, "they have shuffled us nursing students into a room where someone has died." I was frozen entirely until the lead nurse came in and walked to her bedside to wake her up so she could start pushing. That was my first experience seeing a woman with epidural anesthesia. There is nothing wrong with epidurals; it is an intervention that can be very helpful, but it can build a false belief that giving birth is quiet. It's not. You may need to roar, and that is your birthright.

### MOVE

We are made to move. We are roaming creatures whose bodies work best when we move regularly. You are meant to move in labor and birth, as much as you want to and whenever you need to. Your baby is moving too, finding a way through your pelvis, and you will help your baby do that when you move your body.

Imagine you are in a dance together, both doing your part to find the perfect rhythm. Let your baby's movements remind you to keep moving. Movement during labor is how you and your baby co-create momentum through the pelvis as the uterus contracts. Swing, sway, step, dance, rock, pace, march, squat, twist, lunge, swim, twerk, stretch, lean, shimmy, arch, fold, bend, shake...move.

The best birth spaces have room to move and props for support. Watching women move around instinctively in labor is fascinating; each person will have their unique way, often pausing and deep breathing during a contraction, and then back to moving around. If the dominant media image of a person in labor is sitting in a reclined position on a hospital bed, we need a new imagination for birth.

The baby's descent into the pelvis is connected to the maternal movements. As the uterus gently nudges the baby into the pelvis with the muscular contraction of its fibrous tissue, the spaces between the contractions let the baby make all of the little micro adjustments to turn their heads and glide through the bones of the midpelvis. If a birthing mother is left in one position throughout the entirety of the journey, the natural descent of the baby is much more challenging.

My younger sister's first baby came so fast and so early she was born while I was mid-flight on my way to her. She labored quickly but pushed for hours to meet her first daughter. When I finally arrived at the birth center in tears of joy, she proudly told me her midwife's comment was, "I've never seen someone in so many birth positions during labor." Sure enough, her daughter came into the birth canal at a funny angle, making her descent and pushing more difficult. Her baby did make it out vaginally, with the downside of an adorable smushed little nose that straightened back out in a few weeks. So don't fear labor-inspired gymnastics if your body can handle it. It's your primal body doing its thing, and it is helping your baby on the birth journey.

### STAGES

Labor and birth are divided into three "stages," and it may be helpful to understand them. The first stage starts when you move from early labor into active labor (this could be five minutes or five days. Seriously, it depends on a host of factors). The first stage goes all the way from starting labor until you are fully dilated and ready to push. The second stage is the pushing part, and the third stage is the time after the baby is born until your placenta emerges. When you see the phrase "fully dilated," it simply means the biggest part of the baby's head is fully through the dilated cervix (the bottom segment of your uterus) and has moved into the birthing canal (your vaginal opening). At the max stretch point of the cervix (think of a tight turtleneck getting stretched over your ears) and before the head is entirely into the vaginal canal is a very intense time called "transition," the move from first stage (labor) to second stage (pushing). It can be a focused, vivid moment and sometimes requires awareness and an energetic shift.

Labor is a lot of sensation, but it's also passive. Each contraction wave comes to you at a pace and intensity you are responding to and receiving with movement, breathing, noises, and energy. Each "contraction" shortens the muscle fibers of the uterus and, by default, then stretches the cervix around your baby's head. Labor is also rhythmic, with intense waves of sensations around one minute in duration, followed by several minutes of full release and calm. At the peak of the wave, breathing in and out deeply helps you move through the sensation, and when it's fully released, your breath comes back to normal, and your body releases endorphins.

When you come through transition and the baby's head moves through the cervix into the birth canal, there is a shift from passive to active energy. You begin to sense the active downward movement of your baby and may even feel this in your body as an instinct to grunt or bear down as your baby's head moves into the birth canal. Transition is the space for you to go from receiving your contractions to actively joining your contractions with effort (pushing). Making the transition from receiving to "doing something" with each contraction is a part of the journey for you to spend time thinking about and preparing for.

### PUSH

I emphasize the importance of the moment you go from fully dilated to pushing with a personal story.

After decades of providing hands-on midwifery care, I moved into a clinical leadership position in 2021. Shifting into a new career role in healthcare, I knew it was vital for me to spend time with Pamela on The Farm. It was a wonderful visit to mark this huge personal transition. Pamela had just officially retired from delivering babies at 81 years old (how stunning!) and was full of wisdom and support for my transition.

In awe of her years of being with women and her dedication to teaching young midwives, I asked this question: "What is it you share with younger midwives you think is most important?" She answered me very quickly and with passion, "Be patient." She went on to explain that impatience during transition can lead to problems with pushing. "Birthing women are being asked to push before they are ready; the best thing she can do is breathe through those last contractions…this is a spiritual place where she becomes the mother."

Let this sink in. One of the most pioneering midwives in the United States said this was the most critical moment for birth and presence. Let's go back to the media image again: blue gown, lying on a hospital bed now with legs in stirrups and gowned strangers hovering around a vagina to deliver a baby.

This is *not* the way it has to be. The pushing part (second stage) depends on you taking an active role in helping your baby out. The uterus is contracting, but now you are using your "bearing down" reflex, which is something you can usually feel in your pelvis when the baby's head comes into the birth canal (your vagina). Pushing involves your diaphragm and your belly muscles working with each contraction (we all use the diaphragm for strength and leverage daily to perform routine activities, mostly unconsciously). The combination of the muscular uterus and the mother's bearing down reflex nudges that baby's head into the birth canal, and the baby's shoulders follow through the pelvic bones. The best hope you have of all that going well, with or without anesthesia, is that you start when you are fully ready and that you are patient.

For most of us, pushing takes time. Changing positions many times for the duration of the descent is helpful. Between each push, you'll get a few minutes to gather your breath, sip water, feel the love and energy in the room, and center yourself for the next push. And guess what? If you're tired and overwhelmed and just need a moment, you don't have to push at every contraction! Like a surfer ready to ride a wave at the right moment, you can let the perfect moment come and go and not jump up. You'll know when the moment is right, and the next wave is coming.

I had a chance to meet with Ina May Gaskin and show her around a birth center I had helped develop. In her early eighties at the time, she loved the big open rooms with large beds, spacious walk-in showers, and deep soaking tubs. "This is wonderful, Margaret. There is so much room for a mom to move." Ina May told me she wanted the world to learn a new word: *uprightability*. I laughed out loud because I knew exactly what she meant. Upright positions favor the best chances for all the forces and physics of labor to work synergistically. It was something The Farm midwives knew well and actively guided women toward.

Take time imagining this. Think about the positions that might feel good: standing, kneeling, squatting, side-lying, in the water, on your hands and knees. Any position you can conjure up can work with support. If the baby's head has to pass through a space between your pubic bone in the front and the sacrum in the back, any position that collapses this opening (like sitting or lying on your back) may make the pushing part longer. If this isn't making sense, find an image of the pelvis and study it. You'll understand quickly that Ina May's idea of uprightability makes a lot of sense. Uprightability optimizes birth physiology.

In my birth preparation, I had visualized myself pushing side-lying in a bed, so when it came time for me to start pushing my first baby out, that is where I started. When that didn't seem to be working, I tried a birth stool and then stood up for a while. Weary from the energy output, my midwife suggested

I get back into the birth tub and relax for a while. This is what Pamela meant by her wisdom: "Be patient."

I was floating in the tub, trying to rest, but bearing down a little when I *felt* my baby's head move down during a contraction. It was such a relief to feel progress that I stayed right where I was floating in that tub and had a very peaceful (although not planned) water birth.

Let's reimagine how we birth our babies.

**LOVE MATTERS**

Love matters when you labor and push your baby out. Feeling love for yourself and your incredible body, being loved by those in the room, sending loving energy to your baby...all of this lovingkindness supports you in this moment of change.

No matter your spiritual beliefs, lovingkindness is its own practice. It's the sincere wish for oneself and others to be happy, peaceful, and free from suffering, without expectation or attachment. It's a boundless and unconditional love. It's not too much to ask for; it's ancient wisdom to which we are all connected. Consider lovingkindness a bridge that carries you through the transformation. Consider that your birth attendants keep this loving environment consistently strong for you. You can have the most beautiful room, the most tech-advanced equipment, and the most experienced providers, but just as important as all of those things is lovingkindness.

It is the presence of those who love and care for you that will give you strength and comfort on this journey. Oxytocin has been dubbed "the love hormone" in the scientific world, and guess what the dominant hormone of labor is? Oxytocin. Love matters.

Attending a strong young woman at the hospital who was getting ready to push, the room was packed: nurses, techs, nursery staff, family, and friends gathered around her. It was time to push, and she was gathering her strength. No one was coaching her; there was a quiet, silent agreement to take her cues when she was ready. With her head resting back and eyes closed, her face changed slightly, and I knew the next contraction was coming. She opened her eyes, smiled, and said, "I love all of you," and in unison, without rehearsing, we all said back to her in a chorus, "We love you!" She started laughing and pushed her baby out. It brought tears to my eyes.

We were all connected and feeling the beautiful human blueprint.

YOU ARE ENOUGH.

THE HUMAN BLUEPRINT IS BEAUTIFUL.

# homecoming

*"It's not just the birth of a baby,*
*it's the birth of a mother."*

*– Pamela Hunt, The Farm Midwife*

**WELCOME**, you have left the waiting space of expectancy and moved into a time of receiving what you have worked so hard for, the sweet embrace of new life. You may be reading this still pregnant or a partner waiting to meet the baby, and that's OK. Please do enter into your imagination of this time with curiosity and hope. The moment you come face to face with this mysterious little person and receive their sweet presence earthside will stay etched in your consciousness forever. You have come through the passage of conception, pregnancy, labor, and birth into the new parenting identity. This is the best part, the soft landing. Use that breath to ground yourself, receive, and take it all in. Sound dreamy? It is, and it can also come with other emotions like profound fatigue or shock. I've been there to see a person push a baby out and then say to me,

"I feel too weak to hold him." It's OK. Take a moment if you need to, or crack a joke. As I coached a mom to reach down and join my hands to deliver her baby, she brought him to her chest and said, "Oh my goodness, I just gave birth to my husband." The truth was that the baby *did* look just like his dad. We all had a good laugh. Another mom had one girl and then several boys in succession. She promised her daughter, who wanted a sister, that she could get a puppy if this last one were a boy. As I coached her to help bring this baby boy to her chest, the first thing the kiddo heard his mom say was, "Well, sister is getting a puppy."

## BIRTH OF A MOTHER

While this moment of welcoming new life is timeless, in the modern era, we have named it "matrescence,[16]" the birth of a mother. For most of human history, mothers lived in a community and had round-the-clock help after giving birth. The concept of matrescence only emerged in the late 20th century because in our pre-modern era, it was part of part of everyday life. It didn't need its name. Mothers were surrounded with help, and giving birth was the next rite of passage following menstruation. The community came together to ensure each little human and their parents had what they needed. This wasn't something we achieved independently. It was how we survived communally.

---

[16] Raphael, D. (1975). Matrescence, becoming a mother, a "new/old" rite de passage. In *Being female: Reproduction, power, and change* (pp. 65–71). De Gruyter

Modern parenting life has too often isolated us from this treasure of community and support, to our detriment. Today's parents frequently go home to inconsistent support systems, inadequate parental leave, and a mountain of new things to learn. You are *not* supposed to know how to "do it all" while projecting a fabulous, brave image — a false construct from a disconnected world (often reinforced by social media and advertisers).

You should get to be your true self, loved and cared for in community and with complete vulnerability. Modern postpartum community looks different, but I am encouraged by the popularity of postpartum groups, stroller groups, postnatal yoga, and parent get-togethers. We need more sharing, more laughter, more rallying support, and more normalization of the idea that we are communal creatures making an incredible life transition that is made better in connection with each other.

### BONDING

Being skin to skin with your baby is essential to their development. In the womb, the baby gets its first foundation of neuronal growth by absorbing all of the sensory inputs of the mother's body: a steady heartbeat, acoustic sounds, and the rhythmic movement of the body's activities. At the time of birth, these sensory inputs of the newborn are centered in their "primitive" brain. Conditioned by these experiences, newborns are primed to be soothed by rhythm, the distinct tones of the parents' voices, and the movement of the human body. Their first experiences outside the womb send familiar messages to their body and brain: warmth, touch, and tone.

Newborns don't have a strong cognitive function, but they feel everything. Remember the conversation about your brain's three layers? Your baby is born only operating in that lower, reptilian (primitive) layer: sleeping, eating, and eliminating. With each sensory input (your touch, your voice, your gaze, your energy), your baby is building their wiring in the emotional and rational layers of the brain. Most early human connection starts in this same realm of the nonverbal; our feelings come first, and then our thoughts. Love, connection, and emotional warmth through this physical, sensory contact are the beginning pathways for the baby to emotionally regulate, sending an instinctual message of safety and security. Skin-to-skin parent contact after birth isn't a "nice to have," it is an essential ingredient for your baby to thrive. If your little one needs help breathing right after delivery or goes into the intensive care unit, that, of course, is the top priority, and your golden hour for connection starts when you finally have your baby on your body, skin to skin.

#### MILK

How you choose to feed your baby is your decision. In Ali Wong's 2018 Netflix special, "Hard Knock Wife," she's on stage, pregnant with her second baby, and in a leopard print dress, proclaims, "A lot of women have anxiety about giving birth. Well, let me tell you something, giving birth ain't nothing... compared to *breastfeeding*." I remember cackling.

I share this not to instill fear of breastfeeding, but to let you know that it's OK not to be OK if breastfeeding is hard for you. It was hard for me; my midwife ego, which was certain I would know how to do this, felt like it had been backed over by a huge truck. It took me months to figure out a rhythm. Many hospitals provide fantastic lactation consultants; ask for one. If one is unavailable through your provider, I recommend interviewing some so you have options for support. Many communities also have free lactation groups for expert help. If you struggle in the beginning, it does not mean you can't do this. Have them on speed dial as soon as you need help. And contrary to some imagined world where we just hold the baby to our breast and they magically start to nurse, you will probably need help. It's part of the journey.

Please know this: The warm milk your body creates even before your labor begins is full of heroic nutrients and good bacteria that will positively impact your baby's whole life. As a baby lies on the parent's skin and latches to the breast, a message is sent to the brain alerting the body to send the milk. There is emerging evidence that the baby's saliva on the breast signals the mother's body for the particular nutrients and calming molecules the baby needs.[17] How miraculous! Any of this incredible contact and transformative milk will be beneficial to helping you and your baby get off to a great start. If you can't nurse and you can pump, go for it. If you need donor milk to get started, say yes. Don't think twice about it.

---

[17] La Leche League International. (n.d.). *Concept explanations*. https://llli.org/about/policies-standing-rules/psr-concept-explanations/

Some women have *too much* milk supply and donate it. It's not weird. The milk is carefully screened for use, and it's part of a long tradition of women supporting women. Human milk sharing has existed across cultures for centuries. If you feed your baby another way, snuggle your baby while bottle feeding. The connection built in holding and feeding your baby is more than just nutrition; it is wiring their brand-new nervous system with resilience.

### PRACTICING PRESENCE

You may need time to process your experience of giving birth. Take that time. Processing your birth can be very powerful and integral to healing your parts, especially if it did not unfold the way you had expected. As my career developed, I saw how the stories we tell ourselves are sometimes not the things that happened. The brain is very interesting in this way; human memory is notoriously imperfect. Ask for time to sit and debrief your birth with your support people; they may have more to add to the story that might be helpful for you. Birth debriefing was something I came to see over time as very powerful. Processing with the people who attended your birth allows you to align your memory and meaning-making with what unfolded. This is a big part of understanding the story and sometimes the healing.

I remember sitting down to debrief with a young couple who welcomed their first baby with me at the birth center. She had a beautiful labor that was complicated at the very end, so an ambulance was called to transfer her to the hospital.

The intelligence of her body kicked in as we waited for the ambulance, and she made rapid progress. Her baby's head was crowning as the medics were setting up her stretcher, and every person in the room smiled as a gorgeous, pink baby girl let out a big, lusty cry right there at the birth center, moments from being put on a stretcher. With her baby in her arms and the risk averted, she got to recover beautifully in the birth center. As we unpacked this dramatic birth scene and shared our memories weeks later, I got to tell her how strong and powerful she was to me. Tears filled her eyes, and I knew I was in the presence of her healing parts of herself.

Writing about your birth is another good option. We write slower than we think, so writing your birth story on paper slows your thinking and allows reflection and processing to begin. Journaling, writing your birth story, or even writing a letter to your child are all ways to move through the feelings. No matter what unfolded, going back over the details and recording them can open up places inside of you for healing or gratitude, or both. It took me many years to do this for my own experiences, and that might be true for you too, but I can attest to its transformative power.

These activities may feel like an add-on post birth, but trust me, they are essential, and you won't regret it. Make space for processing your journey. Consider this a final way to be present for yourself as this pregnancy and birth chapter ends and your parenting journey begins.

**NESTING**

Bringing your little person home, or sharing your home if that is where they were born, is a treasure. It is hard to capture this time with words because each experience is unique. My parents brought me home to an army tent in the Tennessee woods at the height of the summer in 1974, and I turned out okay. I took my first child home to a tiny apartment in Seattle with a charming view of a parking lot. The families I cared for often wanted to talk to me about what gear or stuff they needed for their baby. I would smile and nod, sometimes offering an idea, but would always remind them of this: what your baby needs most is you, the loving caregiver. With love and support in your home, you will get off to a great start. You need to be confident in this: All feelings are welcome, and all entry points are honored.

Unlike the nesting you did for yourself in labor, this side of nesting brings an added challenge: You need to get to know your baby. They all arrive with different hard-wired temperaments, but none with a handbook. Nesting in this setting means experimenting with your environment to see what brings your baby into calm, and therefore what brings you into precious rest.

Life's rhythms now will likely have no pattern. This is where the beginner's mind you learned in the first trimester comes in handy. Each day is a new beginning, an experiment, and a way to learn about your baby human. I did this four times and parented four different ways. Old formulas or ideas get swapped out with new data inputs from your baby. Yes to rocking, but hates the car seats. Yes to swaddling, no to cold wet wipes at 3:00 a.m. Everything, I mean everything, becomes new, and without good support, a loving community, and a sense of humor, you can get overwhelmed fast.

When I finally arrived at my younger sister's house after her fast-and-furious birth, she told me they wanted to take the night and snuggle as a family. Of course, they did; it was their first tiny baby, and I knew exactly where they were. No less than 30 minutes after bedtime, she woke me in the guest room, handed me her newborn, and said, "I'm not a hero. I need sleep." I loved her openness to an abrupt change of plans and cherished those newborn cuddles with my niece, safely tucked in my arms, skin to skin. I felt proud of my sister for honoring her exhaustion and claiming the rest she needed. We've laughed many times about her saying "I'm not a hero" and embracing vulnerability.

#### RECEIVING HELP

Joy, gratitude, and exhilaration can be mixed with anxiety, fear, depression, and profound exhaustion. You can feel all that in 20 minutes; the ups and downs are normal. As we are a multitude of parts, we all come to mothering in various ways. Just as joy is not always the default emotion when you see a positive pregnancy test, happiness is not always the dominant emotion after birth.

Your placenta, a nice source of all kinds of hormones, is no longer in your body, and whether you choose to breastfeed or not, a new set of hormones is directing your body to make milk for this little person. This abrupt change is a lot for your body (and brain) to go through and can leave you feeling fragile and disembodied.

You will learn (hopefully) from your healthcare providers that the hormonal slump that comes after birth is expected and has a name: the postpartum blues. You will also learn (hopefully) from your healthcare providers that if you start to feel down and don't get better, you could be suffering from postpartum depression. Marked by feelings of sadness, anxiety, and emotional disconnection, the rates for the U.S. are on the rise and disproportionately affecting women of color.[18] Professional organizations are recognizing that women need more than a six-week check-up, but instead close follow-up in the days and weeks after birth to ensure they are not suffering from untreated depression.[19] If it crosses *your* mind at any point, or if you are a partner and it's crossing your mind that what you are experiencing is not garden-variety stress, book a timely appointment to talk to your provider, and if that is not possible, get them on the phone or in a telehealth visit. You need to talk through your experience and may need helpful medical interventions.

Research also suggests that "proximity of neighbors" can decrease rates of depression.[20] This is a modern scientific

---

[18] Khadka, N., Fassett, M. J., Oyelese, Y., Mensah, N. A., Chiu, V. Y., Yeh, M., Peltier, M. R., & Getahun, D. (2024). Trends in postpartum depression by race, ethnicity, and prepregnancy body mass index. *JAMA Network Open*, 7(11), e2446486.

[19] American College of Obstetricians and Gynecologists. (2018). *Optimizing postpartum care*. https://www.acog.org/clinical/clinical-guidance/committee-opinion/articles/2018/05/optimizing-postpartum-care

[20] Onyewuenyi TL, Peterman K, Zaritsky E, et al. Neighborhood Disadvantage,

reflection of the core idea of primitive gynecology. We survived as a species because we helped each other. Receiving help in community is a connection to our early beginnings. You may not be able to magically conjure up friendly neighbors. In that case, it's OK, but please hear this: Making connections, big or small, in any realm of community within your life can positively impact this transitional experience.

Even if we must let modern science rename this as the "neighbor effect," its impact is the timeless truth woven through this book: We need each other on this journey. Early parenting is hard, but it's not impossible, especially when we go through it together. That's how we make it through. That's how we choose to do it again. Most people struggle with these shifts, and this doesn't mean you are not a good parent; this simply means you are human and need your community. Asking for help means you are an incredible parent.

Hormonal changes, major life shifts, and sleep deprivation can combine into a challenging landscape. Talking to your provider during the first days and weeks is a good start. Be very gentle with yourself as you figure things out. Some people sail through this, and others need layers of help and sometimes even medical intervention. Mental health during pregnancy and postpartum is finally getting the attention it deserves, and parents are thankfully less afraid to identify that they are struggling; this is important progress.

---

Race and Ethnicity, and Postpartum Depression. *JAMA Netw Open.* 2023;6(11):e2342398.

Resist the temptation to analyze or judge yourself. It is not helpful or necessary. Wherever you are on this continuum, you are not alone. When stress, fatigue, and anxious thoughts overwhelm you, take a deep breath and exhale slowly. You always have your breath and can calm your system. You are enough; this was always true. You need your community of support more than ever before, and it is here that the power of presence becomes a lifeline.

Deep into my career, and when the last of my four children knew how to put on his velcro shoes, I squeezed into the last seat of a "lunch and learn" about postpartum obsessive-compulsive disorder. A local therapist had come to teach our team about this common but misunderstood disorder. The speaker was excellent, and as I sat there eating my lunch and listening to her lecture, I felt my insides turn over. I had experienced the feelings of the "parent" she was describing. I had some of the symptoms on her bulleted PowerPoint, and I had navigated it alone and insecurely. It was humbling and eye-opening. How many highly functional people are in the throes of mothering and second-guessing everything? So many. Welcome! You are not alone; we *all* need to know that. What must you do if you are worried, disturbed, or afraid? Ask for help and know that you are not alone.

#### HELPFUL HELP

A word here about getting help at home in the early days: Similar to off-handed comments in pregnancy about your changing body catching you off guard, sometimes postpartum help is not helpful. I noticed a pattern when I would do home visits on new mothers fresh from giving birth: A post-childbirth mother would be doing things in the house as per usual, and visitors would be holding the baby. This is a cherished moment for sure, but seriously? Can we change this culturally? Exposure to outside germs is not ideal for the baby, and the idea of the new parents hosting a viewing ritual is terrible for a mother's recovery. The parents should bond with the baby, and the loving community should be mopping, doing laundry, or making a meal. There is plenty of time to hold the baby in the weeks ahead. Postpartum mothers who have had scant hours of decent sleep don't need to be hosting guests and watching them hold their baby. A good rule of thumb should be that if you're still bleeding (which is common for several weeks after birth), you should be off your feet.

A trend is emerging that I applaud: Parents are asking friends to leave meals in a cooler on their porch and posting a list of practical things they need from the store: toilet paper, milk, and fresh fruit. Yes! This is how to be helpful for new parents; baby holding can come later. If you have trouble with boundaries, try saying, "We're focusing on rest and recovery right now, but your help is welcome in other ways. We plan to have visitors start coming by in the next six weeks. Thank you so much for your care. We'll be sure to share some newborn pictures soon." Anyone who cares, or is one of your people, will understand this reasonable request. This is helpful help.

**YOUR STORY**

Becoming a parent elicits strong emotions, both positive and trepidatious. There are a large number of us who had happy childhood experiences, but many of us did not, and some of us have weathered trauma and suffering. A significant group of people arrive at the threshold of parenting, *having never cared for a baby.* It's OK if you are one of these people! There is so much to learn about yourself and this new family member. No matter how you enter parenting, you will be impacted by the metamorphosis. Our relationships with *parenting* are all different and can impact our ideas of *becoming parents.*

Do you feel a sense of fear or inadequacy about this transformation? Does your partner? Welcome, you are in good company. Take a deep breath, trust yourself. You have been allowed to receive something new. This journey is yours now. You can reframe your relationship to parenting simply by honoring who you are right now.

The most important thing you can do when facing inadequacy or insecurity is to ask for and receive help. It sounds easy, but it can be challenging. Rugged American individualism, a cultural narrative pounded into us from the start, suddenly goes head to head with a new reality: You need community. You need people to bring you things and take the sibling to the park so you can nap when the baby sleeps. You need someone to mow your yard, buy diapers, or take your dog on a walk. You need that meal, that baby food, that box of pads. You need help, and you need to be able to access it without an existential crisis.

If we all changed our expectations of what it means to be *with each other* on this journey, it wouldn't feel so cringy. So here is our invitation. Let's remember the embodied truth from our past; we need community and to be *with each other* on this journey.

### YOU ARE BECOMING

Remember earlier in the book when we discussed facing your fears and bringing the power of presence to the forefront? You have everything it takes for this journey, and I am confident in you.

As you begin to identify the moments in your life that matter, the rites of presence in rhythm with your new life, may you continue to use what you have learned: Remember how strong you are, stay rooted in what you know is true, release what does not serve you, and receive support from your community.

A young mother whom I have known since she was a little girl, and one who did not always see eye to eye with her mom, shared her journey of becoming a parent. Her reflections capture so well this beautiful metamorphosis:

*I was raised by an incredible mother, one who taught me the meaning of unconditional love, presence, and nurturing. For me, this journey isn't necessarily about breaking generational cycles. It's been more about deepening my awareness and expanding our roots. It's about being fully present in every moment, breathing through the challenges, and building a home full of love, security, and joy, one moment at a time.*

You get to *create* this next chapter of your life, harnessing what you want (or don't want) from your past and making something new that works for your life. In this sense, you are entering the new world of parenting, a time of transformation where you bring all the tools you have gained and all the wisdom you have developed to begin the inspiring and humbling journey of parenthood.

When you feel lost or overwhelmed, return to the rites: Remembering, Rooting, Releasing, and Receiving.

I hope you are surrounded by loved ones and a community of support on your journey. I hope you will know how to create this for someone, too. The dream is that we build a support system for new families, embracing the joy and the privilege of serving each other through this transformation. This is how humans have survived for thousands of years — in community, in presence with each other. May we reclaim this connected way of living, and may we all share in this privilege of loving connection with ourselves and each other.

May we all bring love into the room.

*"And so may a slow wind work these words of love around you, an invisible cloak to mind your life."*

*– John O'Donohue*

# acknowledgments

**IT IS A TRUE PRIVILEGE TO BE A MIDWIFE.** I have been transformed through sharing sacred spaces with people on sacred journeys. I have witnessed human miracles, allowing me to see how profoundly strong and capable we all are. I have been transformed through witnessing the power of presence. I have been blessed by wise midwives who showed me the power rooted in loving kindness and presence, sharing wisdom and traditions that reshaped my life.

Many incredible people helped me on this journey, so please allow me to honor some of them in order of their appearance. To my parents, of course, thank you for your brave decision to put your lives on a unique path and welcome me earthside into a loving community. Thank you to Pamela Hunt for her loving patience and support as my teacher, and to all of the Farm Midwives who have invested in the next generation of midwives. Thank you to Aretha and Nicole, who helped me believe in myself as a writer, and to Megan, Hannah, Heather, Catherine, Leigha, Chanille, Taneesha, and Johanna who gave me encouragement and feedback. Thank you to Jackson and William, who have always had my back, and to my four children, Lila, Ava, Mack, and Bodie, who are love to me in every room.

Thank you to my *true teachers*, the brave families I have been privileged to serve. You taught me through your vulnerability about the power of presence; you showed me what the truest self was capable of, and I stand in awe of your power. You are the truth-tellers in this book, and I am humbled and grateful to have been part of your journey.

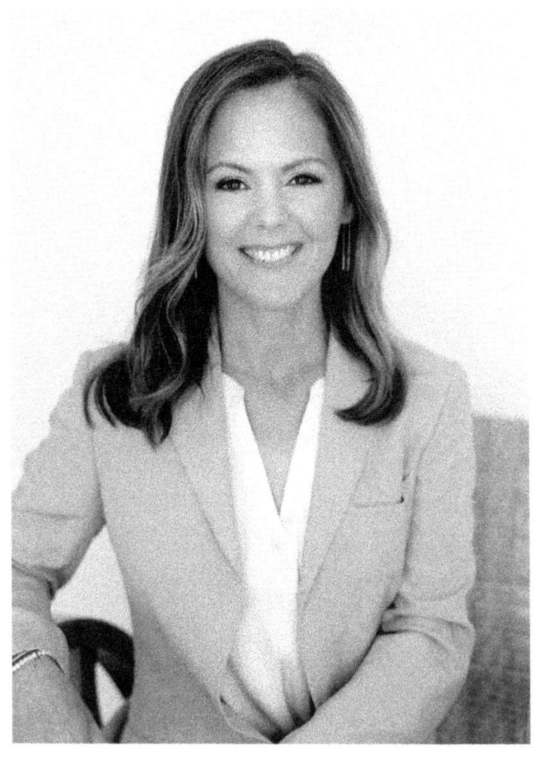

Dr. Margaret Buxton is a Certified Nurse Midwife and passionate advocate for evidence-based, high-value maternity care that extends the range of women's health and birth options within caring, empowered environments. Margaret is a graduate of the Vanderbilt Nurse-Midwifery Program and has a doctorate in nursing from the University of Alabama. Margaret lives and works in Nashville, Tennessee. When she's not working, Margaret loves great food, travel, and spending time with her four children.

www.ingramcontent.com/pod-product-compliance
Lightning Source LLC
LaVergne TN
LVHW021155160826
845679LV00024B/2126